T0362464

Multiple Ligament Knee Injuries

Editors

BRUCE A. LEVY
BENJAMIN FREYCHET

CLINICS IN
SPORTS MEDICINE

www.sportsmed.theclinics.com

Consulting Editor
MARK D. MILLER

April 2019 • Volume 38 • Number 2

ELSEVIER

1600 John F. Kennedy Boulevard • Suite 1800 • Philadelphia, Pennsylvania, 19103-2899

http://www.theclinics.com

CLINICS IN SPORTS MEDICINE Volume 38, Number 2
April 2019 ISSN 0278-5919, ISBN-13: 978-0-323-71218-7

Editor: Lauren Boyle
Developmental Editor: Donald Mumford

Clinics in Sports Medicine (ISSN 0278-5919) is published quarterly by Elsevier Inc., 360 Park Avenue South, New York, NY 10010-1710. Months of issue are January, April, July, and October. Business and Editorial Offices: 1600 John F. Kennedy Blvd., Ste. 1800, Philadelphia, PA 19103-2899. Customer Service Office: 3251 Riverport Lane, Maryland Heights, MO 63043. Periodicals postage paid at New York, NY and additional mailing offices. Subscription prices are $364.00 per year (US individuals), $698.00 per year (US institutions), $100.00 per year (US students), $405.00 per year (Canadian individuals), $861.00 per year (Canadian institutions), $235.00 (Canadian students), $475.00 per year (foreign individuals), $861.00 per year (foreign institutions), and $235.00 per year (foreign students). Foreign air speed delivery is included in all *Clinics* subscription prices. All prices are subject to change without notice. **POSTMASTER:** Send address changes to *Clinics in Sports Medicine*, Elsevier Health Sciences Division, Subscription Customer Service, 3251 Riverport Lane, Maryland Heights, MO 63043. Customer Service (orders, claims, online, change of address): Elsevier Health Sciences Division, Subscription Customer Service, 3251 Riverport Lane, Maryland Heights, MO 63043. **Tel: 1-800-654-2452 (U.S. and Canada); 314-447-8871 (outside U.S. and Canada). Fax: 314-447-8029. E-mail: journalscustomerservice-usa@elsevier.com (for print support); journalsonlinesupport-usa@ elsevier.com (for online support).**

Reprints. For copies of 100 or more of articles in this publication, please contact the Commercial Reprints Department, Elsevier Inc., 360 Park Avenue South, New York, NY 10010-1710. Tel.: 212-633-3874; Fax: 212-633-3820; E-mail: reprints@elsevier.com.

Clinics in Sports Medicine is covered in *MEDLINE/PubMed (Index Medicus) Current Contents/Clinical Medicine, Excerpta Medica,* and *ISI/Biomed.*

Contributors

CONSULTING EDITOR

MARK D. MILLER, MD
S. Ward Casscells Professor, Head, Department of Orthopaedic Surgery, Division of Sports Medicine, University of Virginia, Charlottesville, Virginia, USA; Team Physician, Miller Review Course, Harrisonburg, Virginia, USA

EDITORS

BRUCE A. LEVY, MD
Professor, Department of Orthopedic Surgery and Sports Medicine, Mayo Clinic, Rochester, Minnesota, USA

BENJAMIN FREYCHET, MD
Department of Orthopedic Surgery and Sports Medicine, Mayo Clinic, Rochester, Minnesota, USA

AUTHORS

CHRISTOPHER P. BANKHEAD, MD
PGY-IV, Resident, Department of Orthopaedic Surgery, University of New Mexico, Albuquerque, New Mexico, USA

AARON BEACH, PhD
Sydney Orthopaedic Research Institute (SORI), Chatswood, New South Wales, Australia

ANDREW BERNHARDSON, MD
The Steadman Clinic, Vail, Colorado, USA

JOEL BOYD, MD
Associate Professor, Department of Orthopaedic Surgery, University of Minnesota, Minneapolis, Minnesota, USA

PATRICK S. BUCKLEY, MD
The Steadman Clinic, Vail, Colorado, USA

JOHN DABIS, MBBS, MRCS, FRCS (Tr&Orth) MSc, SEM
Sports Knee Fellow, Brisbane Orthopaedic & Sports Medicine Centre, Queensland, Australia

VISHAL S. DESAI, BS
Departments of Orthopedic Surgery and Sports Medicine, Mayo Clinic, Rochester, Minnesota, USA

WESLEY BRADLEY DOSHER, MD
Resident Physician, Department of Orthopaedic Surgery, The University of Texas Health Science Center at Houston, Houston, Texas, USA

LARS ENGEBRETSEN, MD, PhD
Oslo University Hospital, University of Oslo, OSTRC, Norwegian School of Sports Sciences, Oslo, Norway

GREGORY C. FANELLI, MD
Geisinger Orthopaedics, Danville, Pennsylvania, USA

BENJAMIN FREYCHET, MD
Department of Orthopedic Surgery and Sports Medicine, Mayo Clinic, Rochester, Minnesota, USA

AARON GIPSMAN, MD
Department of Orthopaedic Surgery, Keck Medical Center of the University of Southern California, Los Angeles, California, USA

CHRISTOPHER D. HARNER, MD
Professor, Department of Orthopaedic Surgery, The University of Texas Health Science Center at Houston, Houston, Texas, USA

JARRED K. HOLT, DO
Fellow, Orthopaedic Sports Medicine and Shoulder, Tria Orthopaedic Center, Bloomington, Minnesota, USA

MITCHELL I. KENNEDY, BS
Steadman Philippon Research Institute, Vail, Colorado, USA

NICHOLAS I. KENNEDY, MD
Departments of Orthopedic Surgery and Sports Medicine, Mayo Clinic, Rochester, Minnesota, USA

AARON J. KRYCH, MD
Departments of Orthopedic Surgery and Sports Medicine, Mayo Clinic, Rochester, Minnesota, USA

ADAM KWAPISZ, MD, PhD
Orthopaedic Surgery, Pan Am Clinic, University of Manitoba, Winnipeg, Manitoba, Canada; Clinic of Orthopedics and Pediatric Orthopedics, Medical University of Lodz, Lodz, Poland

ROBERT F. LAPRADE, MD, PhD
The Steadman Clinic, Vail, Colorado, USA; Complex Knee and Sports Medicine Surgery and Adjunct Professor, Orthopaedic Surgery, University of Minnesota, Minneapolis, Minnesota, USA; Affiliate Faculty, College of Veterinary Medicine and Biomedical Sciences, Colorado State University, Fort Collins, Colorado, USA

BRUCE A. LEVY, MD
Department of Orthopedic Surgery and Sports Medicine, Mayo Clinic, Rochester, Minnesota, USA

ADAM LINDSAY, MD
Department of Orthopaedic Surgery, Keck Medical Center of the University of Southern California, Los Angeles, California, USA

PETER MACDONALD, MD, FRCSC
Orthopaedic Surgery, Pan Am Clinic, University of Manitoba, Winnipeg, Manitoba, Canada

NIV MAROM, MD
Hospital for Special Surgery, New York, New York, USA

ROBERT G. MARX, MD
Hospital for Special Surgery, New York, New York, USA

GRAEME MATTHEWSON, MD
Orthopaedic Surgery, Pan Am Clinic, University of Manitoba, Winnipeg, Manitoba, Canada

GARRETT T. MAXWELL, BS
Medical Student, The University of Texas Health Science Center at Houston, McGovern Medical School, Houston, Texas, USA

GILBERT MOATSHE, MD, PhD
Oslo University Hospital, University of Oslo, OSTRC, Norwegian School of Sports Sciences, Oslo, Norway

DARLI MYAT, PhD
Sydney Orthopaedic Research Institute (SORI), Chatswood, New South Wales, Australia

NORIMASA NAKAMURA, MD, PhD
Institute for Medical Science in Sports, Osaka Health Science University, Osaka City, Osaka, Japan

THOMAS NERI, MD, PhD
Sydney Orthopaedic Research Institute (SORI), Chatswood, New South Wales, Australia

DAVID ANTHONY PARKER, BMedSci, MBBS, FRACS, FAOrthA
Sydney Orthopaedic Research Institute (SORI), Chatswood, New South Wales, Australia

DUSTIN L. RICHTER, MD
Assistant Professor, Director of Sports Medicine Research, Department of Orthopaedic Surgery, University of New Mexico, Albuquerque, New Mexico, USA

GEORGE F. RICK HATCH, MD
Department of Orthopaedic Surgery, Keck Medical Center of the University of Southern California, Los Angeles, California, USA

THOMAS L. SANDERS, MD
Departments of Orthopedic Surgery and Sports Medicine, Mayo Clinic, Rochester, Minnesota, USA

TRENY SASYNIUK, MSc
Orthopaedic Surgery, Pan Am Clinic, University of Manitoba, Winnipeg, Manitoba, Canada

ROBERT C. SCHENCK Jr, MD
Professor, Chair, Department of Orthopaedic Surgery, University of New Mexico, Albuquerque, New Mexico, USA

MICHAEL J. STUART, MD
Departments of Orthopedic Surgery and Sports Medicine, Mayo Clinic, Rochester, Minnesota, USA

NICHOLAS A. TRASOLINI, MD
Department of Orthopaedic Surgery, Keck Medical Center of the University of Southern California, Los Angeles, California, USA

GEHRON P. TREME, MD
Associate Professor, Program Director, Department of Orthopaedic Surgery, University of New Mexico, Albuquerque, New Mexico, USA

ANDREW VEITCH, MD
Associate Professor, Head Team Physician, Department of Orthopaedic Surgery, University of New Mexico, Albuquerque, New Mexico, USA

RYAN J. WARTH, MD
Research Program Manager, Department of Orthopaedic Surgery, The University of Texas Health Science Center at Houston, Houston, Texas, USA

DANIEL C. WASCHER, MD
Professor, Division Chief, Sports Medicine, University of New Mexico, Albuquerque, New Mexico, USA

ADRIAN WILSON, MBBS, MRCS, FRCS (Tr&Orth)
Professor, Consultant Knee and Sports Surgeon, The Wellington and Portland Children's Hospitals, London, United Kingdom

Contents

The knee dislocation is a severe, complex injury that can be difficult to treat and is fraught with complications. The first step in a successful reconstruction of a multiple ligamentous knee injury is gaining an accurate and thorough understanding of the pattern of instability imparted by the injury. Evaluation begins with a detailed review of radiographic and advanced imaging studies followed by a thorough physical examination, often done under anesthesia, in conjunction with dynamic fluoroscopy. Failure to identify and reconstruct a damaged ligament may place undue stress on adjacent structures, resulting in complications and potential failure of the surgical procedure.

Classification systems should enhance communication between providers, facilitate accurate and consistent reporting in the literature, and guide management. However, current classification systems for MLKIs lack sufficient detail to guide clinical management which limit their prognostic value. The purpose of this chapter is to revisit and consider important features of some of the most impactful classification systems developed in the orthopaedic literature and to propose a classification system for MLKIs that may improve communication among providers, facilitate consistent reporting in the literature, and ultimately foster publication of meaningful clinical data.

The multiple ligament injured knee (knee dislocation) is oftentimes part of a multisystem injury complex that can include injuries not only to knee ligaments but also to blood vessels, skin, nerves, bones (fractures), head, and other organ system trauma. These additional injuries can affect surgical timing for knee ligament reconstruction and also affect the results of treatment. This article presents the author's approach and experience to the initial assessment and treatment of the multiple ligament injured (dislocated) knee.

plan. Surgical repair and reconstruction of the involved ligaments are frequently discussed in the literature; however, osteotomy to correct limb malalignment may be just as important to obtaining a good outcome. Limb realignment must be carefully evaluated and treated. Isolated soft tissue procedures are prone to failure if significant malalignment, deformity, and thrust are ignored. In select cases, osteotomy can lead to restored mechanical stability, optimal joint load distribution, improved survival of simultaneous soft tissue procedures, and better patient outcomes.

CLINICS IN SPORTS MEDICINE

SERIES OF RELATED INTERESTED

Orthopedic Clinics
Foot and Ankle Clinics
Hand Clinics
Physical Medicine and Rehabilitation Clinics
Clinics in Podiatric Medicine and Surgery

THE CLINICS ARE AVAILABLE ONLINE!
Access your subscription at:
www.theclinics.com

Foreword

Multiple Ligament Knee Injuries: Expert Insight

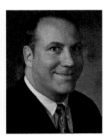

Mark D. Miller, MD
Consulting Editor

Multiple ligament knee injuries (MLKI) are often very challenging and require experience, a keen knowledge of anatomy, and dedicated surgeons to properly manage. I have been fortunate to belong to an international cadre of knee surgeons who share a similar interest in this topic. Although there is no formal MLKI study group, this same group of surgeons has contributed numerous Instructional Course Lectures, Symposia, scientific sessions, publications (including this issue of *Clinics in Sports Medicine*), and even a Department of Defense–sponsored research effort: the STaR project that is now underway.

This issue of *Clinics in Sports Medicine* was put together by my good friend Bruce Levy, who is one of the leaders of the MLKI group. He has invited international experts to provide insight in the diagnosis, classification, and management of these complex injuries. As Dr Levy points out, each MLKI is different, so it is helpful to have a broad understanding of this topic. This issue of *Clinics in Sports Medicine* is a great start.

Mark D. Miller, MD
Division of Sports Medicine
Department of Orthopaedic Surgery
University of Virginia
James Madison University
400 Ray C. Hunt Drive, Suite 330
Charlottesville, VA 22908-0159, USA

E-mail address:
mdm3p@virginia.edu

https://doi.org/10.1016/j.csm.2019.01.002
0278-5919/19/© 2019 Published by Elsevier Inc.
sportsmed.theclinics.com

Preface

Knee Multiligament Injury

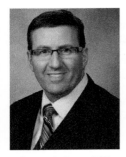
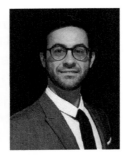

Bruce A. Levy, MD   Benjamin Freychet, MD

Editors

Managing multiple ligament knee injury (MLKI) can be quite complex. Optimal treatment strategies are evolving but significant strides have been made with regards to surgical technique leading to improved patient reported outcomes. No two MLKIs are the same, and each patient requires an individualized approach. Controversies persist with regards to repair versus reconstruction of injured ligamentous structures, early versus late surgical management, and early versus delayed rehabilitation. Because these patients and their knee injury patterns are so heterogeneous in nature, it is difficult to perform high-level research to answer these highly debated questions.

In this issue of *Clinics in Sports Medicine*, we have brought together a group of international experts who have demonstrated a clinical interest and have published extensively in this field. Although level 1 randomized clinical trials are rare for this type of injury, level 5 evidence can actually provide significant insights into the optimal management of the MLKI.

The studies that have been compiled for this symposium focus on the importance of clinical diagnosis for ligament injury patterns, malalignment, meniscus, cartilage, and neurovascular injury. The authors present their preferred techniques for ACL and PCL reconstructions and MCL and LCL surgery, including when to repair and when to reconstruct.

Clin Sports Med 38 (2019) xv–xvi
https://doi.org/10.1016/j.csm.2019.01.001
0278-5919/19/© 2019 Published by Elsevier Inc.

This issue is addressed to orthopedic residents, fellows, and practicing surgeons searching for guidance on treatment of the MLKI based on the best available evidence in 2019.

Bruce A. Levy, MD
Department of Orthopedic Surgery and Sports Medicine
Mayo Clinic
200 First Street Southwest
Rochester, MN 55905, USA

Benjamin Freychet, MD
Department of Orthopedic Surgery and Sports Medicine
Mayo Clinic
200 First Street Southwest
Rochester, MN 55905, USA

E-mail addresses:
Levy.Bruce@mayo.edu (B.A. Levy)
benjamin.freychet@gmail.com (B. Freychet)

Knee Ligament Instability Patterns: What Is Clinically Important

Joel Boyd, MD[a],*, Jarred K. Holt, DO[b]

KEYWORDS

- Multiligamentous knee injury • Knee dislocation • Knee instability

KEY POINTS

- The initial evaluation of a complex, multiligamentous knee injury begins with a systematic and thorough physical and radiologic evaluation to determine the precise nature of instability about the joint.
- Evaluation includes review of advanced imaging, which is then correlated with physical examination, often under anesthesia, along with dynamic fluoroscopy to confirm the site involved, direction, and severity of the instability imparted by the injury.
- The major structures about the knee that are most often disrupted include the anterior cruciate ligament, posterior cruciate ligament, and either the medial collateral ligament or posterolateral corner complex; occasionally all 4 ligamentous restraints are injured.
- Failure to identify a concomitant injury may jeopardize the outcome of the surgical reconstruction; as such, it is important to accurately determine the clinically important patterns of instability and develop a comprehensive surgical plan.

INTRODUCTION

The first step in successfully treating the multiple ligament injured knee is the performance of a thorough, accurate evaluation to recognize the degree and pattern of ligamentous instability about the joint. A comprehensive understanding of the anatomy, biomechanics, and injury patterns allows the treating surgeon to develop a focused surgical plan to restore stability. The identification and correction of medial and lateral instability is paramount to performing successful reconstruction of the cruciate ligaments, because these structures work synergistically to stabilize the joint. Using a

Disclosure Statement: Drs J. Boyd and J.K. Holt have no relevant financial disclosures related to the authorship of this work.
a Department of Orthopaedic Surgery, University of Minnesota, Minneapolis, MN, USA;
b Orthopaedic Sports Medicine and Shoulder, Tria Orthopaedic Center, 8100 Northland Drive, Bloomington, MN 55431, USA
* Corresponding author.
E-mail address: Joel.Boyd@Tria.com

Clin Sports Med 38 (2019) 169–182
https://doi.org/10.1016/j.csm.2018.12.001
0278-5919/19/Crown Copyright © 2019 Published by Elsevier Inc. All rights reserved.

multitude of diagnostic tools, including advanced imaging, examination under anesthesia, and fluoroscopic stress images, the treating surgeon will be able to identify clinically important ligamentous instability and develop an appropriate, comprehensive surgical reconstruction plan.

In 1992, Schenck and colleagues developed their classification describing the typical ligamentous injuries associated with knee dislocations (**Fig 1**). This descriptive classification identifies which of the 4 major ligamentous structures about the knee have been disrupted. It has been modified several times, now to include letter designations including those injuries with an associated fracture (V), those with associated arterial injury (C), and those with associated nerve injury (N).[1] In general, a classic traumatic knee dislocation involves a Schenck type III or IV injury, typically requiring disruption of the both the anterior and posterior cruciate ligaments (PCLs) along with at least one collateral structure to produce a full dislocation. KDIIIM and KDIIIL injuries are the most common patterns resulting in true articular dislocation.[2] An isolated cruciate with concomitant collateral injury rarely imparts enough soft tissue instability to result in frank joint incongruity, although dislocations with unicruciate injuries have been described previously.[3] In addition to using the Schenck anatomic classification to gain an initial understanding of the ligament injury, an understanding of the direction of displacement of the tibia with respect to the femur at the time of the initial evaluation can also predict the individual structures damaged. Kennedy[4] described his positional classification of knee dislocations, categorizing the injury

Anatomic Classification of Knee Dislocations			
Schenck 1992			
I	single cruciate + collateral	ACL + collateral	
		PCL + collateral	
II	ACL / PCL	collaterals intact	
III M	ACL / PCL / MCL	LCL+PLC intact	
III L	ACL / PCL / LCL+PLC	MCL intact	
IV	ACL / PCL / MCL / LCL+PLC		
V	fracture dislocation		
C	arterial injury		
N	nerve injury		

Fig. 1. Schenck classification of knee dislocations. ACL, anterior cruciate ligament; LCL, lateral collateral ligament; MCL, medial collateral ligament; PCL, posterior cruciate ligament; PLC, posterolateral corner.

based on the location of the tibia relative to the femur. Although this is a well-established and useful descriptive classification it may be difficult to apply in all cases, because it has been purported that up to 50% of knee dislocations spontaneously reduce before the initial evaluation.

A number of studies support the notion that anterior dislocations of the knee occur most commonly, followed closely by posterior injuries.[4–6] In a large review of 245 cases, it was noted that 40% of knee dislocations presented with the anterior displacement of the tibia relative to the femur.[5] This is most often caused by a severe hyperextension mechanism, resulting in failure of the posterior capsule, PCL, and anterior cruciate ligament (ACL). Posterior dislocations accounted for approximately 33% of injuries in their cohort, typically owing to a direct blow to the anterior proximal tibia on a flexed knee, as often occurs in the so-called dashboard injury. Occult dislocations more commonly occur with a combination of lateral, medial, and rotatory forces, often as a result of indirect injury. Direct lateral and medial dislocations are relatively uncommon, comprising approximately 18% and 4% of knee dislocations.[5] Particular attention should be payed to the direct lateral or posterolateral dislocation in the emergent setting as the medial femoral condyle may buttonhole through the medial capsule, interposing tissue into the joint and rendering closed reduction quite difficult or impossible.[7]

Advanced imaging is the diagnostic modality of choice for injury characterization following initial emergency room management. MRI provides the ability to identify the location of injuries, degree of ligament disruption, integrity of the adjacent soft tissue envelope, and evaluate bony and articular surfaces. It has demonstrated to be up to 100% sensitive and specific in characterizing ligamentous injury about the knee.[8] In conjunction with MRI, a comprehensive physical examination allows the surgeon to further identify the pattern and degree of instability. Owing to the nature of the injury, a physical examination in the clinical setting is often severely limited, as such a thorough examination under anesthesia is crucial. A thorough examination of the knee includes evaluation of each of the major ligamentous periarticular structures to characterize the degree of instability imparted by the injury. Dynamic fluoroscopic evaluation is also of substantial benefit to confirm ligamentous instability. The examination is used to confirm clinically important patterns of instability, which are previously suggested by findings of advanced imaging and to develop the final plan of surgical reconstruction.

ANTERIOR INSTABILITY

Injury to the ACL is commonly encountered in the setting of knee dislocation, occurring in up to 90% of multiligamentous injuries.[9] The location of ACL disruption is quite variable; it has been reported that in 32% of cases an intraligamentous rupture is seen, whereas 24% of cases demonstrate femoral-sided avulsion and 26% are tibial-sided avulsions.[10] Femoral or tibial avulsions with bony fragments are quite rare, more often occurring as tibial spine fractures in the pediatric population. Disruption of the ACL results in loss of restraint to anterior tibial translation as well some of degree of loss of rotational control. It is now well-accepted that the posterolateral bundle of the ACL plays a significant role in restraint to internal rotation of the tibia, along with a number of other periarticular structures.[11,12] Clinically significant instability is easily evaluated in a similar manner to those patients with isolated ACL disruption, namely, via the Lachman maneuver, anterior drawer test, and pivot-shift phenomenon. In the setting of a multiligamentous injury, especially those with combined PCL and medial meniscus injury, anterior tibial translation becomes quite exaggerated. This finding can be confirmed with dynamic anterior drawer fluoro-scopic analysis.

POSTERIOR INSTABILITY

The PCL can be considered the keystone to ligamentous stability of the knee in the face of multiligamentous injuries. It has a multifaceted biomechanical role that, when disrupted, results not only in significant sagittal translation, but also in rotational and coronal plane instability. In the intact state, it essentially provides a central pivot point for the knee; however, when disrupted, this allows for multiplaner translation resulting in substantial instability and risk for frank dislocation. It has been demon-strated that PCL disruption is noted in 79% to 87% of all knee dislocations, with the large majority of these injuries occurring at the proximal insertion midsubstance.[9,10] Similar to disruption of the ACL, distal avulsion injuries with or without bony fragments have been described as well; these injuries must be identified, because they may be amenable to primary repair rather than reconstruction[13–15] (Fig 2). In a series of 63 knee dislocations Twaddle and colleagues[8] noted that 51% of identified PCL injuries were considered amenable to primary reattachment.

Clinical evaluation of the PCL begins with an understanding of the complex biome-chanical role of the structure. As the largest of the intraarticular ligaments, the PCL provides the majority of restraint to posterior tibial translation at all flexion angles and contributes 95% of posterior stability of the tibia between 30° and 90° of flexion.[16] Similar to the ACL, the PCL is a 2-bundled unit consisting of a separate anterolateral and posteromedial bundles, which are defined based on their location of attachment at the medial femoral condyle. The anterolateral bundle is quite larger and stiffer than the anteromedial, comprising 85% of its cross-sectional area.[16] Previous studies sup-ported the notion that the majority of posterior translation stability was conferred by the larger anterolateral bundle[17]; however, recent work suggests a more codominant role between the bundles, especially at flexion angles of greater than 90°.[18] It has also been noted through sectioning studies that, in the fibular collateral ligament (FCL) intact state, the PCL provides little varus restraint; however, when the FCL is deficient the PCL becomes the key secondary stabilizer to varus force.[19,20] Additionally, the PCL plays a key secondary role in restraint to external rotation of the tibia in conjunc-tion with the posterolateral complex.[21]

Examination of the PCL injured knee is begun with simple observation of the resting posture of the knee at 90° of flexion. In the case of significant PCL instability the sag sign is easily noted as the tibial plateau is pulled posteriorly by gravity, result-ing in the loss of abnormal contour of the anterior knee. In a resting position, the plateau should sit anterior to the distal aspect of the femoral condyles. A posterior drawer testing in this position elicits further posterior instability in the PCL-deficient knee as well. It has been documented that posterior drawer testing is approximately 90% sensitive and more than 99% specific for the identification of PCL injury and subsequent posterior instability.[22] Often in the case of the multiliga-mentous knee injury substantial, gross posterior translational instability of more than 15 mm will be seen; this is felt to be indicative of combined PCL and posterolateral corner (PLC) disruption. Last, performance of the dial test, in which the injured knee is subjected to external rotation force at both 30° and 90° of flexion is carried out and compared with the uninvolved, contralateral side. A side-to-side difference of greater than 10° external rotation with the knee at 90° suggests PCL insufficiency, whereas increases in rotation 30° indicate PLC laxity and increases at both 30° and 90° sug-gest combined PCL–PLC laxity.[23]

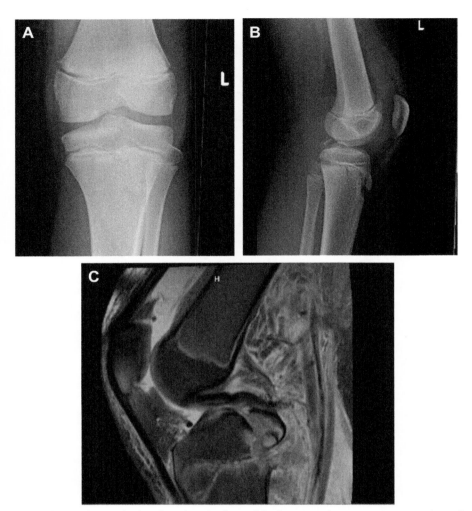

Fig. 2. Plain radiographs (*A*, *B*) and sagittal MRI (*C*) of patient demonstrating comminuted tibial-sided posterior cruciate ligament avulsion in a 12-year-old boy. This injury was amenable to primary repair.

The physical examination findings of posterior instability can then be further confirmed with dynamic fluoroscopic evaluation. This evaluation is done by first obtaining a true lateral fluoroscopic view of the knee at rest at 90° of flexion. Often with gross instability there will be radiographic evidence of the sag sign at this resting position. With the addition of a manually imparted posterior drawer gross incompetence of the PCL and secondary restraints to posterior tibial translation will be evidenced by further posterior translation of the tibial plateau (**Fig 3**).

MEDIAL AND POSTEROMEDIAL INSTABILITY

The ligamentous anatomy of the medial side of the knee is described as having 2 distinct structures, the medial collateral ligament (MCL) and posteromedial corner

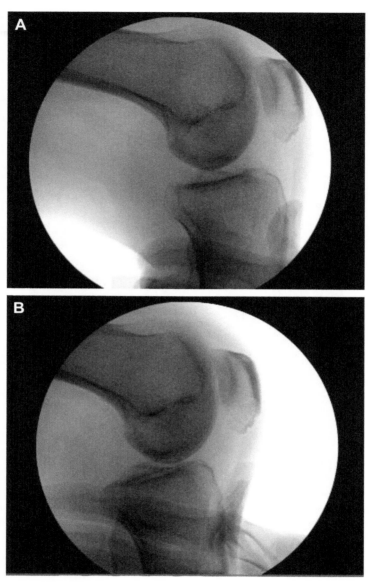

Fig. 3. Dynamic fluoroscopic posterior drawer demonstrating posterior translation of the tibial plateau in the posterior cruciate ligament (PCL)-deficient knee. (*A*). Knee in neutral position (*B*). Knee with posterior force applied. Note the significant posterior translation of the tibia indicative of PCL insufficiency.

(PMC) complex. The MCL is a thick, taut blending of 3 individual structures, the superficial MCL, the deep MCL, and the posterior oblique ligament (POL). The superficial portion of the MCL complex originates from a depression just posterior and proximal to the medial epicondyle and terminates with a long, broad attachment to the proximal tibia approximately 6 cm distal to the joint line.[24] In contrast, the deep MCL is more of a longitudinal thickening of the capsule with distinct meniscofemoral and meniscotibial attachments.[25] The POL is a separate, distinct structure lying posterior to the superficial MCL, inserting onto the margin of the articular surface, the posterior joint capsule, and blending into the semimembranosus tendon.[24] The entire MCL complex is dynamically reinforced by the pes anserinus tendons; collectively the POL, capsule, oblique popliteal ligament, and pes tendons are termed the posterior medial corner (PMC).

The superficial MCL provides primary restraint to valgus stress across all knee flexion angles, with the deep fibers acting as a secondary stabilizer.[26] Particularly, it has been noted that the anterior fibers of the superficial MCL impart much of the restraint to valgus stress.[27] The MCL also acts as a secondary restraint to anterior tibial translation in the ACL-deficient knee; it has been noted that the MCL experiences a nearly 300% increase in peak force during walking after sectioning of the ACL.[28,29] Competence of the MCL is evaluated with valgus stress testing performed at 30° of flexion, with disruption manifested as greater than 5 mm of medial joint opening. This same maneuver shoulder be performed at 0° of flexion as well; in this position, the POL and PMC also have been shown to provide restraint to valgus stress, along with contributions of the cruciates.[30] Instability at 30° followed by relative stability with the maneuver at 0° is indicative of isolated MCL disruption, whereas instability at both is concerning for combined loss of valgus and posteromedial rotational control. It is important to note that, when performing this maneuver, the knee must be maintained in external rotation. As with evaluation of posterior instability, valgus incompetence can be confirmed with similar maneuvers performed in conjunction with dynamic fluoroscopy as well.

The PMC complex encompasses a number of structures, including the POL, oblique popliteal ligament, joint capsule, meniscotibial ligaments, and semimembranosus tendon. The PMC complex acts in conjunction with the MCL as a restraint to valgus force in extension, but slackens during flexion.[31] More important, the PMC, specifically the POL, plays a key role preventing rotational instability. When disrupted the medial tibial plateau rotates around the axis of the PCL, resulting in posteromedial translation. The PMC complex is assessed by coupling internal rotation with posterior drawer testing at approximately 90° of flexion. It should be noted that, in combined PMC and PCL injury, rotational instability may be more difficult to discern as typically the tibia rotates around the intact fibers of the PCL. When disrupted this, axis is lost and the tibia inherently lies in a posteriorly subluxed position without a fulcrum for rotational motion.

Injury patterns at the medial knee can be quite variable in location as disruption has been noted at the femoral insertion, midsubstance, and distal insertion sites. Distal injuries to the MCL are of most concern owing to retraction and development of a Stener-type lesion, which is felt to preclude healing without surgical treatment (**Fig 4**). In a study of 28 multiligamentous knee injuries with medial sided involvement it was discovered that 14 of these injuries were distal avulsions, 5 proximal avulsions, and remainder midsubstance disruptions.[8] In their series, the investigators identified that 68% of medial-sided injuries were considered reattachable ligamentous avulsions based on MRI findings, indicating that close scrutiny of the location of the lesion should be undertaken and consideration given for primary repair of a subset of these injuries.

LATERAL AND POSTEROLATERAL INSTABILITY

The anatomy of the lateral side of the knee, similar to the medial side, is quite complex and involves a number of structures, each with varying roles in conferring stability to the knee joint. Although multiple individual structures have been identified at

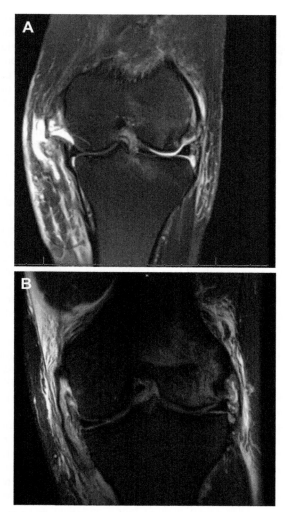

Fig. 4. MRI of medial collateral ligament (MCL) injuries. (*A*). Coronal MRI demonstrating a full-thickness, femoral-sided tear of the MCL with retraction from its insertion adjacent to the medial epicondyle. (*B*). Coronal MRI demonstrating full-thickness distal MCL injury with retraction. The location and retraction of the injury resulted in a Stener-type lesion of the ligament with respect to the pes anserinus tendons.

the PLC, the 3 most important components are that of the FCL, popliteus tendon, and popliteofibular ligament. The FCL, similar to the MCL, arises from a small depression proximal and posterior to lateral epicondyle and runs distally approximately 70 mm to insert directly onto the fibular head approximately 28 mm anteroinferior to the fibular styloid tip.[32] The popliteus muscle originates from the posteromedial proximal tibia and runs laterally, becoming tendinous at the popliteal fossa and inserting 18.5 mm anterior and distal to the proximal origin of the FCL.[32,33] A continuation of the popliteus tendon, the popliteofibular ligament consists of an anterior and larger posterior band, both of which insert on the proximal fibular styloid.[20,32]

Mechanically, the PLC complex is primarily responsible for conferring restraint against varus stress, external tibial rotation, and also plays a role in controlling posterior translation.[15] The FCL is the primary stabilizer to varus stress across all angles of flexion, although its greatest role occurs at 0° to 30° of flexion.[20] The remainder of the PLC, along with the PCL, assume a greater role at greater flexion angles. These structures, particularly the popliteus and popliteofibular ligament, also provide restraint to posterolateral rotation of the tibia. It has been demonstrated through progressive sectioning that the PLC structures resist external rotation at early angles of flexion, particularly the LCL at 0° to 30° and the popliteus and popliteofibular ligament at higher degrees.[34] At 90° of flexion, the PCL takes over to confer external rotation stability; these findings are the foundation of the dial test described previously.[19] Additionally, the PLC corner also plays a secondary role in preventing posterior translation in conjunction with the PCL. Those same sectioning studies demonstrated that isolated PCL deficiency results in a maximum of 11 mm of posterior tibial translation whereas combined PCL and PLC disruption results in 15 to 21 mm of displacement. Identification of combined PCL and PLC injury is important to a successful reconstruction; it has been demonstrated that failure to restore PLC integrity may increase the risk for continued PCL instability and graft failure.[35]

Severe, combined injuries to this site result in substantial mechanical instability manifested as severe varus thrust, external rotation, and recurvatum upon physical examination. Observation of increased recurvatum and external rotation when the limb is suspended with the knee in extension is the first clue to injury of the PLC (**Fig 5**). The varus stress, posterolateral drawer, dial, and reverse pivot shift tests all are used clinically to evaluate the degree of instability secondary to PLC disruption. Varus stress testing should be performed at both 0° and 30° of flexion. With isolated LCL disruption only small, sometimes imperceptible to appreciation joint line opening will be discovered; however, with disruption of the deeper PLC structures, significant gapping will be present. Substantial joint line opening with varus stress at 0° is more indicative of a combined, severe injury to the PLC, PCL, and potential ACL, as often seen in KDIIIL type injuries.[33,36] As with medial-sided injury, varus stress under dynamic fluoroscopy is often used to confirm LCL incompetence (**Fig 6**). The dial test, as discussed, is an important maneuver used to further

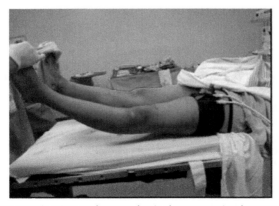

Fig. 5. Preoperative examination under anesthesia demonstrating hyperextension, varus, recurvatum instability of the left lower extremity secondary to a combined posterior cruciate ligament and posterolateral corner injury.

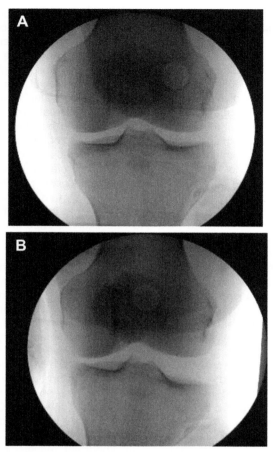

Fig. 6. Dynamic fluoroscopic evaluation of lateral sided ligamentous instability. (*A*). Antero-posterior (AP) fluoroscopic image with knee at neutral position. (*B*). AP fluoroscopic image with varus stress. Note the significant lateral joint opening indicative of fibular collateral ligament injury.

characterize the degree of rotational instability. A 10° increase in external rotation of the tibia at 30° is indicative of isolated PLC injury; however, increases at both 30° and 90° suggest combined PLC–PCL insufficiency. The posterolateral drawer maneuver and its accompanying reverse pivot-shift examination are also used to evaluate for combined posterolateral laxity. The posterolateral drawer is performed with the knee flexed to 90° and the tibia externally rotated. A posterior directed force is induced and external rotation of the lateral plateau relative to the femoral condyle is detected. In the setting of PLC insufficiency, this rotation may be marked; however, in combined PLC and PCL injury the findings may be subtler as the rotation pivot point is lost. The reverse pivot shift is performed in a similar manner, applying an external rotation load in conjunction with valgus stress as the knee is taken from flexion to extension. In the case of PLC incompetence, the lateral tibial plateau will begin subluxed in flexion but reduce beneath the condyle with flexion owing to the pull of an intact iliotibial band.

Isolated injuries to the PLC are somewhat rare; however, in the setting of a multiligamentous disruption, they become quite more pronounced. Consisting of the FCL, popliteus tendon, popliteofibular ligament, fabellofibular ligament, and biceps femoris tendon, disruption of one or all of these structures is seen in approximately 77% of patients with bicruciate injuries.[9] A variety of injury patterns are demonstrated, including isolated femoral-sided FCL injury, isolated popliteus injury, or a combination thereof. Distally, disruption of the FCL insertion at the fibula has been demonstrated, although treating surgeons must be vigilant for avulsion injuries of the biceps tendon, termed the "arcuate" fracture. These avulsions are quite common, occurring in up to 88% of distally based PLC injuries.[8] A classification system has been developed to describe the location and concomitant injuries associated with PLC disruption (**Fig 7**). A type I injury is defined as an isolated ligamentous injury at the femoral insertion of a PLC structure, including the FCL, popliteus, and PFL. A type IIa injury is a combined ligamentous injury to the distal FCL in conjunction with the biceps femoris with avulsion or fracture of fibular head. Type IIb is a combined injury to the PLC at its proximal origin,

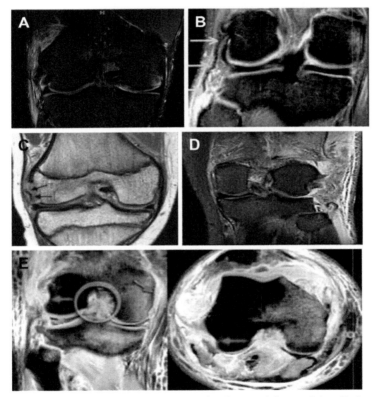

Fig. 7. Boyd classification of posterolateral corner (PLC) injury. (*A*) Type I injury (isolated fibular collateral ligament [FCL] disruption). (*B*) Type IIA combined injury of FCL with hamstring at proximal fibula. (*C*) Type IIB combined injury of FCL and popliteus at femoral origin. (*D*) Type IIIA, severe injury involving FCL, popliteus, and capsule at proximal femoral insertion. (*E*) Type IIIB combined injury of PLC and cruciates. *Arrows* in (*B*): fibular sided FCL + hamstring avulsion injury. *Arrows* in (*C*): note femoral avulsion of popliteus tendon. *Blue and Red arrows* in (*E*): combined disruption of FCL and popliteus tendon. *Green arrow* in (*E*): note concomitant femoral sided MCL injury. *Yellow circle* in (*E*): complete disruption of both cruciate ligaments.

rather than distal. A type IIIa injury is a more severe variant with varying combinations of disruption of the FCL, popliteus, biceps femoris, capsule, and IT band, whereas type IIIb indicates this same injury in conjunction with unicruciate or bicruciate disruption.

SUMMARY

The management of the multiple ligament knee injury is quite complex. Maximizing success and optimizing outcomes of these patients must begin with an accurate and thorough characterization of the individual instability pattern. Although classification systems have been developed to simplify this process, each injury should be treated with an individualized approach. Failure to identify a concomitant injury may significantly jeopardize the functional outcome of the knee as a whole; as such, it is imperative that all ligament instability patterns be identified and addressed at the time of surgical reconstruction. The use of advanced imaging, fluoroscopic stress views, and careful examination under anesthesia will limit these mistakes and aid in restoration of function to the multiple ligament injured knee.

REFERENCES

1. Wascher DC. High-velocity knee dislocation with vascular injury. Treatment principles. Clin Sports Med 2000;19:457–77.
2. Becker EH, Watson JD, Dreese JC. Investigation of multiligamentous knee injury patterns with associated injuries presenting at a level I trauma center. J Orthop Trauma 2013;27(4):226–31.
3. Bratt HD, Newman AP. Complete dislocation of the knee without disruption of both cruciate ligaments. J Trauma 1993;34(3):383–9.
4. Kennedy JC. Complete dislocation of the knee joint. J Bone Joint Surg Am 1963; 45(5):889–904.
5. Green NE, Allen BL. Vascular injuries associated with dislocation of the knee. J Bone Joint Surg Am 1997;59:236–9.
6. Gustilo RB, Cabatan DM. Traumatic dislocation of the knee. St Louis (MO): Mosby; 1993.
7. Quinlan AG, Sharrard WJ. Postero-lateral dislocation of the knee with capsular interposition. J Bone Joint Surg Br 1958;40(4):660–3.
8. Twaddle BC, Hunter JC, Chapman JR, et al. MRI in acute knee dislocation. J Bone Joint Surg Br 1996;78(4):573–9.
9. Becker EH, Watson JD, Dreese JC. Investigation of multiligamentous knee injury patterns with associated injuries presenting at a level I trauma center. J Orthop Trauma 2013;27(4):226–31.
10. Richter M, Bosch U, Wippermann B, et al. Comparison of surgical repair or reconstruction of the cruciate ligaments versus nonsurgical treatment in patients with traumatic knee dislocations. Am J Sports Med 2002;30(5):718–27.
11. Andersen HN, Dyhre-Poulsen P. The anterior cruciate ligament does play a role in controlling axial rotation in the knee. Knee Surg Sports Traumatol Arthrosc 1997; 5(3):145–9.
12. Gabriel MT, Wong EK, Woo SL, et al. Distribution of in situ forces in the anterior cruciate ligament in response to rotatory loads. J Orthop Res 2004;22(1):85–9.
13. Chen SY, Cheng CY, Chang SS, et al. Arthroscopic suture fixation for avulsion fractures in the tibial attachment of the posterior cruciate ligament. Arthroscopy 2012;28(10):1454–63.

14. Nicandri GT, Klineberg EO, Wahl CJ, et al. Treatment of posterior cruciate ligament tibial avulsion fractures through a modified open posterior approach: operative technique and 12-to 48-month outcomes. J Orthop Trauma 2008;22(5):317–24.
15. Gollehon DL, Torzilli PA, Warren RF. The role of the posterolateral and cruciate ligaments in the stability of the human knee. A biomechanical study. J Bone Joint Surg Am 1987;69(2):233–42.
16. Bowman KF Jr, Sekiya JK. Anatomy and biomechanics of the posterior cruciate ligament, medial and lateral sides of the knee. Sports Med Arthrosc Rev 2010; 18(4):222–9.
17. Markolf KL, Feeley BT, Tejwani SG, et al. Changes in knee laxity and ligament force after sectioning the posteromedial bundle of the posterior cruciate ligament. Arthroscopy 2006;22(10):1100–6.
18. Kennedy NI, Wijdicks CA, Goldsmith MT, et al. Kinematic analysis of the posterior cruciate ligament, part 1: the individual and collective function of the anterolateral and posteromedial bundles. Am J Sports Med 2013;41(12):2828–38.
19. Grood ES, Stowers SF, Noyes FR. Limits of movement in the human knee. Effect of sectioning the posterior cruciate ligament and posterolateral structures. J Bone Joint Surg Am 1988;70(1):88–97.
20. Sanchez AR, Sugalski MT, LaPrade RF. Anatomy and biomechanics of the lateral side of the knee. Sports Med Arthrosc Rev 2006;14(1):2–11.
21. Veltri DM, Deng XH, Torzilli PA, et al. The role of the cruciate and posterolateral ligaments in stability of the knee: a biomechanical study. Am J Sports Med 1995;23(4):436–43.
22. Rubinstein RA Jr, Shelbourne KD, McCarroll JR, et al. The accuracy of the clinical examination in the setting of posterior cruciate ligament injuries. Am J Sports Med 1994;22(4):550–7.
23. Lubowitz JH, Bernardini BJ, Reid JB III. Current concepts review: comprehensive physical examination for instability of the knee. Am J Sports Med 2008;36(3):577–94.
24. LaPrade RF, Ly TV, Wentorf FA, et al. The anatomy of the medial part of the knee. J Bone Joint Surg Am 2007;89(9):2000–10.
25. Brantigan OC, Voshell AF. The tibial collateral ligament: its function, its bursae, and its relation to the medial meniscus. J Bone Joint Surg Am 1943;25(1):121–31.
26. Griffith CJ, LaPrade RF, Johansen S, et al. Medial knee injury. Am J Sports Med 2009;37(9):1762–70.
27. Warren LF, Marshall JL, Girgis F. The prime static stabilizer of the medial side of the knee. J Bone Joint Surg Am 1974;56(4):665–74.
28. Haimes JL, Wroble RR, Grood ES, et al. Role of the medial structures in the intact and anterior cruciate ligament-deficient knee: limits of motion in the human knee. Am J Sports Med 1994;22(3):402–9.
29. Shelbourne KB, Pandy MG, Torry MR. Comparison of shear forces and ligament loading in the healthy and ACL-deficient knee during gait. J Biomech 2004;37(3): 313–9.
30. Marshall JL, Baugher WH. Stability examination of the knee: a simple anatomic approach. Clin Orthop Relat Res 1980;(146):78–83.
31. Robinson JR, Sanchez-Ballester J, Bull AM, et al. The posteromedial corner revisited: an anatomical description of the passive restraining structures of the medial aspect of the human knee. Bone Joint J 2004;86(5):674–81.
32. LaPrade RF, Ly TV, Wentorf FA, et al. The posterolateral attachments of the knee. Am J Sports Med 2003;31(6):854–60.
33. Terry GC, LaPrade RF. The posterolateral aspect of the knee: anatomy and surgical approach. Am J Sports Med 1996;24(6):732–9.

34. LaPrade RF, Tso A, Wentorf FA. Force measurements on the fibular collateral ligament, popliteofibular ligament, and popliteus tendon to applied loads. Am J Sports Med 2004;32(7):1695–701.
35. Harner CD, Vogrin TM, Höher J, et al. Biomechanical analysis of a posterior cruciate ligament reconstruction: deficiency of the posterolateral structures as a cause of graft failure. Am J Sports Med 2000;28(1):32–9.
36. Veltri DM, Warren RF. Instructional course lectures, The American Academy of Orthopaedic Surgeons. Posterolateral instability of the knee. J Bone Joint Surg Am 1994;76(3):460–72.

Multiple Ligament Knee Injuries

Current State and Proposed Classification

Wesley Bradley Dosher, MD[a], Garrett T. Maxwell, BS[b],
Ryan J. Warth, MD[a], Christopher D. Harner, MD[a],*

KEYWORDS

- Multiple ligament knee • Knee dislocation • Complex knee • Classification

KEY POINTS

- An effective classification system will enhance communication between providers, facilitate accurate and consistent reporting in the literature, and guide management protocols to improve patient outcomes.
- The current classification systems for multiligamentous knee injuries do not meet all of these criteria.
- Traditional classification systems provide little information on timing of injury (acute, chronic), grade of injury (partial, complete), details on the specific location of the anatomic structures injured, meniscus and articular cartilage injuries, fracture types (avulsion vs non-avulsion), and details regarding concomitant injuries (skin, tendons, meniscus, and cartilage, among others).

INTRODUCTION

The overall prevalence of multiligamentous knee injuries (MLKIs) has seen a steady rise in the United States over recent years.[1] However, although MLKIs can be simply defined as any injury involving more than one knee ligament, very few MLKIs are clinically, functionally, or prognostically equivalent. Currently, the most frequently used classification system is the anatomically based Schenck classification.[2] Other less-often used classification systems focus on either the direction of dislocation or the level of energy involved in producing the injury.[1,3] Although traditional classification systems provide some details regarding a patient's knee injury, they lack sufficient detail to guide clinical management and thus have limited prognostic value.

Disclosure Statement: The authors have no disclosures.
[a] Department of Orthopaedic Surgery, University of Texas Health Science Center at Houston, 6400 Fannin Street, Suite 1700, Houston, TX 77030, USA; [b] University of Texas Health Science Center at Houston, McGovern Medical School, 6400 Fannin Street, Suite 1700, Houston, TX 77030, USA
* Corresponding author.
E-mail address: Christopher.Harner@uth.tmc.edu

Clin Sports Med 38 (2019) 183–192
https://doi.org/10.1016/j.csm.2018.11.006
0278-5919/19/© 2018 Elsevier Inc. All rights reserved.

The purpose of this article is to give an overview of some existing musculoskeletal classification systems in use, define what we believe are important additional components that should be considered, and provide suggestions for what a "new" classification system for MLKIs may look like.

WHAT MAKES AN EFFECTIVE CLASSIFICATION SYSTEM?

Before we introduce a new classification system, we must first define what components go into an effective classification system. An effective classification system will enhance communication between providers, facilitate accurate and consistent reporting in the literature, and guide management protocols to improve patient outcomes. We have chosen 2 clinically accepted classification systems currently in use as examples.

The Burkhart Classification of Rotator Cuff Tears

The creators of this classification system believe a valuable classification system allows for communication between clinicians and researchers, provides information on treatment and prognosis, and allows for comparison of epidemiologic data and treatment outcomes.[4] The investigators realize the importance of using modern imaging techniques in describing the geometric classification of rotator cuff tears. The system not only describes the various tear patterns, but also suggests treatment options and prognosis for each tear subtype.

The Vancouver Classification of Periprosthetic Femur Fractures

This classification system is based off of reproducible evaluation of plain radiographs that were then validated with intraoperative findings.[5,6] The important feature seen with this scheme is that the classification of fractures was directly used to determine operative intervention, which we believe to be an important aspect of any classification system. The Vancouver system is also easily communicated between clinicians and in the literature.

The list of classification systems in the orthopedic literature is extensive, but for the purposes of this article, the 2 previously discussed classification systems will serve as examples of effective, clinically meaningful classification systems.

CURRENT CLASSIFICATION SYSTEMS
Energy and Velocity

A precise classification of what constitutes high-energy versus low-energy injury has not been directly described in the knee dislocation literature. In general, the literature considers victims of motor vehicle collisions, motorcycle collisions, auto versus pedestrian injuries, and other "high-speed" injuries as "high energy." This is in contrast to the classic use of low energy, which classically has referred to patients who have sporting injuries or sustain a fall from standing.[7]

It is worth taking time to briefly mention the new addition of the "ultra–low-velocity knee dislocation" (ULVKD) described by Azar and colleagues.[8] They use the term to describe dislocations that occur "during activities of daily living, such as stepping off a curb, stepping off a stair, or simply falling while walking." With an ever-growing obese population in the United States, the incidence of ULVKD could see a steady rise. This is important because accurate diagnosis of these injuries can be difficult given their mechanism and challenging physical examination. The consequences of missing these injuries can be catastrophic, given their relatively high vascular and neurologic injury rates.[8]

Directional

The directional classification was described by Kennedy in 1963.[3] The classification system is simple, in that it describes dislocations as anterior, posterior, medial, lateral, or rotatory. Rotatory dislocation can be subclassified as anterolateral, posterolateral, anteromedial, and posteromedial. This system is limited because more half of knee dislocations spontaneously reduce before assessment in the emergency department.[9] The directional classification of dislocations does allow for easy communication between clinicians but fails to provide a prognosis or guide clinical treatment of patients.

Anatomic

The most commonly used classification system is the anatomically based Schenck classification (**Table 1**). The Schenck classification was initially described in 1994, modified by Wascher and colleagues[9] in 1997 to include vascular injuries as well as specify medial versus lateral injuries, and then described in detail in Robert Schenck's 2003 article with the conclusion "Classifying knee dislocation is best performed based on what structures are torn, and use of the anatomic system allows for communication and surgical planning."[2,9,10] Schenck does make the concession at the end of the 2003 article[2] that recommends surgeons take into account the energy of injury, even though his classification system does not directly address this component.

Looking at the anatomic classification system critically, it does fulfill some of the necessary components of an effective classification system and certainly represents a significant improvement of previous classification schemes. The system has in particular allowed for significantly improved communication between providers over the past several decades. However, the classification does still lack the necessary specificity to facilitate accurate and consistent reporting. The most important issue with this system is that it does not consistently guide clinical decision making. This is further illustrated in our case examples at the end of the article.

IMPORTANCE OF STANDARDIZED LITERATURE REPORTING

Performing clinical studies of MLKI with a high level of evidence presents multiple obstacles, including the relative infrequency of the injuries, the wide variety of injury mechanisms and patterns, the lack of a clinically more detailed classification system, and the varied treatment options available to surgeons who manage these injuries. To create a new or modified classification system will require adding additional information to help clinicians make informed decisions on treatment. **Table 2** is a summary of a systematic literature search of the PubMed and EMBASE databases (60 studies) that

Table 1 Modified Schenck classification that is currently used in clinical practice	
Category	**Injury Patterns**
KD-I	ACL or PCL + collateral
KD-II	ACL + PCL
KD-III-M	ACL + PCL + medial
KD-III-L	ACL + PCL + lateral
KD-IV	ACL + PCL + medial + lateral
KD-V	Any MLKI with periarticular fracture

Specifiers: M, medial; L, lateral; N, nerve; C, artery.
Abbreviations: ACL, anterior cruciate ligament; MLKI, multiligamentous knee injury; PCL, posterior cruciate ligament.

Table 2
Reporting frequency of Critical Factors (CFs) reported in the literature relevant to the management of multiligamentous knee injuries across the most commonly declared subtopics

Variables Reported	±Operative	±External Fixation	±Delayed	±Staging	±Collateral Surgery	Repair vs Reconstruction	Graft Selection
Number of studies[a]	5	7	9	9	7	12	2
Age	5	2	7	9	6	11	2
BMI	0	0	1	1	1	1	0
Anticipated noncompliance	0	1	0	0	1	1	0
Neurovascular status	5	5	6	6	3	7	0
Degree of polytrauma	1	2	3	2	1	2	0
Reduction status[b]	0	0	2	1	0	0	1
Injury chronicity[c]	5	7	9	9	7	12	2
Injury grade[d]	2	3	7	6	6	7	2
Injury location[e]	0	0	0	0	0	1	0
Injury type[f]	2	0	2	2	1	4	0
Status of collaterals	4	7	9	8	5	11	2
Presence of fractures	4	4	6	7	2	6	2
Nature of prior knee surgeries	0	0	0	1	0	0	2
Nature of concomitant injuries	3	2	4	5	3	7	1

Most Commonly Reported Subtopics of Interest

Note: Shaded boxes represent CFs specific to the corresponding sub-topics of interest.
[a] N = 60 studies addressed a total of 70 subtopics.
[b] Reported whether the knee had spontaneously reduced on presentation, or whether the knee was reduced on initial radiographs.
[c] Reported breakdown of acute and chronic injuries.
[d] Reported breakdown of partial and complete ligamentous injuries.
[e] Reported location of injury along the length of each ligamentous structure (proximal, mid-substance, distal).
[f] Reported breakdown of soft tissue injuries versus bony avulsion injuries.

we performed to determine the reporting frequency of critical factors that would be necessary for specific clinical decision (eg, operative vs nonoperative, repair vs reconstruction, early vs delayed surgery). The gray boxes represent what we deem to be the 3 most important patient parameters for each question of interest; clearly, there exists wide variability in the frequency of the most important variables. The lack of consistent reporting standards for clinical studies involving MLKIs prevents between-study comparisons, even among groups of studies that attempt to answer the same clinical question. **Table 2** provides some important variables that should be included in future MLKI studies, but can also serve as a guideline from which a new classification system for MLKIs could be constructed.

WHAT SHOULD A NEW MULTILIGAMENTOUS KNEE INJURY CLASSIFICATION SYSTEM INCLUDE?

Using retrospective data from 287 patients who presented to our institution with MLKIs, we evaluated relationships between the current KD (knee dislocation) classification and subsequent management strategies to identify injury characteristics that could predict surgical management (Warth RJ, unpublished data, 2018). We found that the KD classification in isolation was not predictive of the type of surgery performed or the need for staged procedures. We found that surgical management strategies became much more predictable after considering the combinations of structures injured, specifying the grades of ligament injuries, and the specifying the location of medial-sided injuries (proximal, mid-substance, distal). For example, posterior cruciate ligament (PCL) injuries were predictably treated surgically when combined with an anterior cruciate ligament (ACL) injury, partial PCL tears were much less likely to be treated surgically than complete PCL tears, and PCL surgeries were much more likely to be staged when a concomitant lateral-sided injury was present. Medial-sided injuries were significantly less likely to be treated surgically, whereas lateral-sided injuries were predictive of surgical treatment; partial tears involving either the medial or lateral side were more likely repaired primarily, whereas complete tears were more often reconstructed with a graft. We also found that, with respect to medial-sided injuries, distal tears were more likely to undergo suture repair, mid-substance tears were much more likely to be reconstructed with a graft, and proximal tears were more likely to be treated nonoperatively. Surgical staging was predicted by the presence of concomitant fractures (after exclusion of avulsion injuries), nerve injuries, and vascular injuries (**Table 3**). There were no significant relationships between injury timing (acute, chronic) and any of the treatment options analyzed.

FUTURE MULTILIGAMENTOUS KNEE INJURY CLASSIFICATION SYSTEMS

Our retrospective data indicated that the KD classification was not predictive of the treatment provided. Using our data, it becomes apparent that a new classification system should include each specific structure injured (ACL, PCL, medial structures, lateral structures), modifiers for fractures and extensor mechanism injuries, nerve injuries, or vascular injuries, as well as possibly including the specific anatomic location of structures injured (proximal, mid-substance, distal), especially for medial-sided injuries.

One tool that could better illustrate knee ligament injuries is the Müller map.[11] The Müller map would allow for a visual representation of specific structures injured and can be further modified to show specific location and severity of injuries. An example of this can be seen in **Fig. 1**. There would also have to be a place for modifiers with regard to ipsilateral fractures and neurovascular injuries. Although our retrospective

Table 3
Summary of predicted management decisions for specific ligamentous injuries according to logistic regression

Injury Feature	Partial Tear		Complete Tear		Surgery Staging	
	Prediction	Odds Ratio[a]	Prediction	Odds Ratio[a]	Prediction	Odds Ratio[a]
ACL injury	Recon	2.8 (2.0–3.8)	Recon	2.9 (2.1–4.0)	NS	—
PCL injury	Recon or Repair	1.4 (1.4–1.5)	Recon	1.9 (1.7–2.1)	Staged when combined with lateral-side injury	1.3 (1.1–1.5)
Medial-side injury	Repair	1.3 (1.1–1.5)	Recon or Repair	1.4 (1.4–1.5)	NS	—
Proximal	Repair	5.2 (1.7–15.7)	NS	—	NS	—
Mid-Substance	NS	—	Recon	8.9 (1.0–80.2)	NS	—
Distal	Repair	7.1 (2.1–24.5)	Repair	24.7 (5.4–114.2)	NS	—
Lateral-side injury	Repair	1.2 (1.1–1.4)	Recon or Repair	1.4 (1.4–1.5)	Staged when combined with PCL injury	1.3 (1.1–1.5)
Fracture	—	—	—	—	Staged	1.2 (1.1–1.4)
Nerve Injury	—	—	—	—	Staged	1.2 (1.1–1.4)
Vascular Injury	—	—	—	—	Staged	1.4 (1.3–1.6)

Dashes indicate the data field was either not applicable or relevant.
Abbreviations: ACL, anterior cruciate ligament; NS, predictive variables were not statistically significant ($P<.05$); PCL, posterior cruciate ligament; Recon, reconstruction.
[a] All reported odds ratios are statistically significant according to logistic regression analyses; 95% confidence intervals in parentheses.

data did not show a statistically significant difference in the eventual treatment of acute versus chronic injuries, we still feel that this should be included in the classification system, as it represents an important landmark during clinical decision making.

CASE EXAMPLES

Using Muller maps, we have chosen several case examples to better illustrate the potential confusion in classifying MLKIs using the current Schenck classification (**Table 4**).

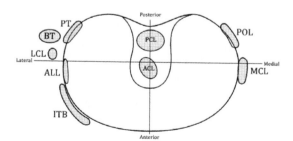

Fig. 1. The Müller map. ALL, Anterolateral Ligament; BT, Biceps Femoris Tendon; ITB, Iliotibial Band; LCL, Lateral Collateral Ligament; MCL, Medial Collateral Ligament; POL, Popliteal Oblique Ligament; PT, Patellar Tendon. (*Adapted from* Müller W. The knee: form and function. Springer-Verlag Berlin Heidelberg: Springer; 1982; with permission.)

Table 4
Common clinical scenarios in which MLKIs are classified into the same KD categories but are treated differently

KD Classification	Injury Pattern Among KD Categories that Require Different Treatment Strategies	Corresponding Müller Map
KD-I	Acute complete ACL tear with complete LCL tear	
	Chronic complete PCL tear with a partial posterolateral corner tear (intact LCL)	
KD-II	Chronic complete ACL tear with partial PCL tear	
	Acute complete ACL tear with complete PCL tear	

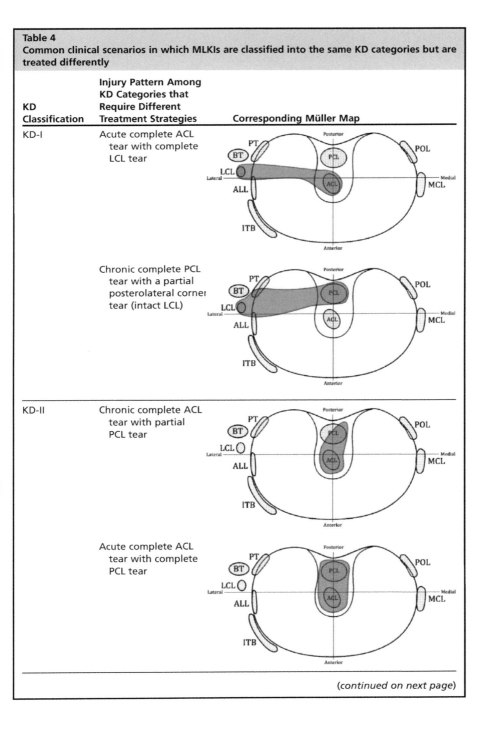

(continued on next page)

Table 4
(*continued*)

KD Classification	Injury Pattern Among KD Categories that Require Different Treatment Strategies	Corresponding Müller Map
KD-III-M	Acute and complete tear of ACL/PCL/MCL	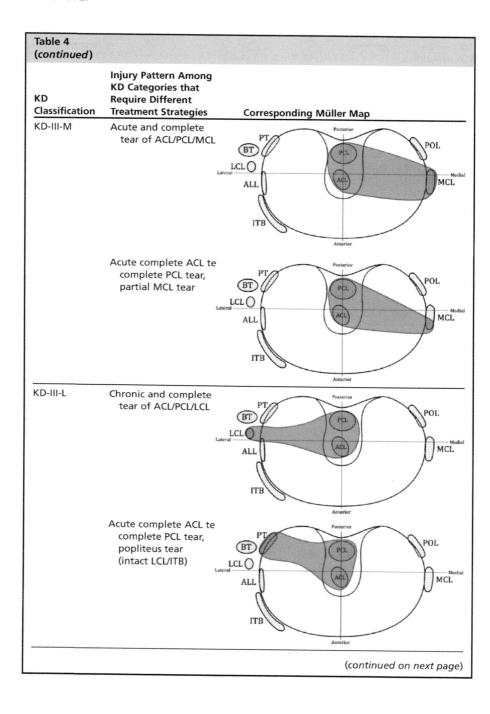
	Acute complete ACL te complete PCL tear, partial MCL tear	
KD-III-L	Chronic and complete tear of ACL/PCL/LCL	
	Acute complete ACL te complete PCL tear, popliteus tear (intact LCL/ITB)	

(*continued on next page*)

Table 4 **(continued)**		
KD Classification	**Injury Pattern Among KD Categories that Require Different Treatment Strategies**	**Corresponding Müller Map**
KD-IV	Chronic complete ACL, complete PCL, complete distal MCL, complete LCL (intact popliteus)	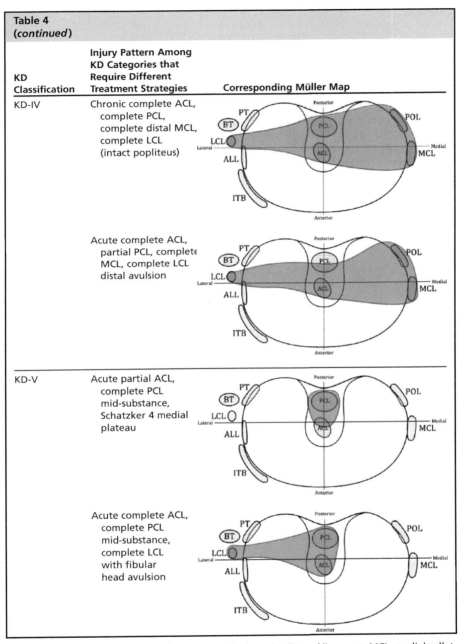
	Acute complete ACL, partial PCL, complete MCL, complete LCL distal avulsion	
KD-V	Acute partial ACL, complete PCL mid-substance, Schatzker 4 medial plateau	
	Acute complete ACL, complete PCL mid-substance, complete LCL with fibular head avulsion	

Abbreviations: ACL, anterior cruciate ligament; LCL, lateral collateral ligament; MCL, medial collateral ligament; MLKI, multiligamentous knee injury; PCL, posterior cruciate ligament.

Adapted from Müller W. The knee: form and function. Springer-Verlag Berlin Heidelberg: Springer; 1982; with permission.

SUMMARY

The use of classification systems to enhance communication between providers, facilitate accurate and consistent reporting in the literature, and guide management protocols to improve patient outcomes remains critical in modern orthopedics. The current MLKI classification system is now more than 20 years old and certainly represents an improvement over previous classification systems; however, it is our hope that by creating a classification system that includes each specific structure injured (ACL, PCL, medial structures, lateral structures), modifiers for fractures, extensor mechanism injuries, nerve injuries, or vascular injuries, as well as specific anatomic location of structures injured meniscus and articular cartilage injuries, and injury timing (acute, chronic) that we can use this information to guide further research in this field and to ultimately improve patient care.

REFERENCES

1. Arom GA, Yeranosian MG, Petrigliano FA, et al. The changing demographics of knee dislocation: a retrospective database review. Clin Orthop Relat Res 2014; 472:2609–14.
2. Schenck R. Classification of knee dislocations. Oper Tech Sports Med 2003;11: 193–8.
3. Kennedy JC. Complete dislocation of the knee joint. J Bone Joint Surg Am 1963; 45:889–904.
4. Davidson J, Burkhart SS. The geometric classification of rotator cuff tears: a system linking tear pattern to treatment and prognosis. Arthroscopy 2010;26:417–24.
5. Duncan CP, Masri BA. Fractures of the femur after hip replacement. Instr Course Lect 1995;44:293–304.
6. Brady OH, Garbuz DS, Masri BA, et al. The reliability and validity of the Vancouver classification of femoral fractures after hip replacement. J Arthroplasty 2000; 15:59–62.
7. Shelbourne KD, Porter DA, Clingman JA, et al. Low-velocity knee dislocation. Orthop Rev 1991;20:995–1004.
8. Azar FM, Brandt JC, Miller RH 3rd, et al. Ultra-low-velocity knee dislocations. Am J Sports Med 2011;39:2170–4.
9. Wascher DC, Dvirnak PC, DeCoster TA. Knee dislocation: initial assessment and implications for treatment. J Orthop Trauma 1997;11:525–9.
10. Schenck RC Jr. The dislocated knee. Instr Course Lect 1994;43:127–36.
11. Müller W. The knee: form and function. Springer-Verlag Berlin Heidelberg: Springer; 1982.

Multiple Ligament Injured Knee

Initial Assessment and Treatment

Gregory C. Fanelli, MD*

KEYWORDS

- Multisystem injury complex • Articular surface • Alignment • Instability pattern
- Vascular assessment • Surgical timing • Staged reconstruction • External fixation

KEY POINTS

- Multiple knee ligament injuries can be part of a multisystem injury complex that can affect treatment outcomes.
- Articular surface fractures must be anatomically reduced and secured before instability patterns can be determined.
- Correction of lower-extremity malalignment with varus or valgus thrust during the stance phase of gait should be considered before ligament reconstruction to optimize results.
- Vascular assessment of both the arterial and the venous systems in the injured lower extremity is important.
- Determination of the instability patterns in the injured knee is important for surgical planning and results optimization.
- Surgical timing for each case may be affected by surgical timing modifiers.

INTRODUCTION

The multiple ligament injured knee (knee dislocation) is oftentimes part of a multisystem injury complex that can include injuries not only to knee ligaments but also to blood vessels, skin, nerves, bones (fractures), head, and other organ system trauma. These additional injuries can affect surgical timing for knee ligament reconstruction and also the results of treatment. This article presents the author's approach and experience to the initial assessment and treatment of the multiple ligament injured (dislocated) knee.

FRACTURES

Articular surface fractures in the multiple ligament injured (dislocated) knee must be anatomically reduced and internal fixation achieved before the knee ligament instability pattern can be determined because the intact femur or tibia will fall into the

Geisinger Orthopaedics, 115 Woodbine Lane, Danville, PA 17822-5212, USA
* 147 Kaseville Road, Danville, PA 17821.
E-mail address: gregorycfanelli@gmail.com

Clin Sports Med 38 (2019) 193–198
https://doi.org/10.1016/j.csm.2018.11.004
0278-5919/19/© 2019 Elsevier Inc. All rights reserved.

fracture and potentially hinder an accurate knee ligament injury diagnosis. Tibial plateau depression fractures that meet nonsurgical criteria with intact knee ligaments should be anatomically reduced and secured because the tendency will be for the femoral condyle to fall into the fracture site, perpetuate the instability, and compromise knee ligament repair or reconstruction.

ALIGNMENT

Femur or tibia fractures requiring reduction and fixation may require that multiple ligament reconstruction be performed after fracture healing has occurred. When varus or valgus alignment with resultant varus or valgus thrust during the stance phase of gait is present after fracture healing, consideration should be given to fracture fixation hardware removal (stage 1) followed by corrective osteotomy (stage 2) to restore normal alignment and gait pattern, followed by knee ligament reconstruction (stage 3) when the osteotomy has healed and osteotomy hardware has been removed if necessary. A normal gait pattern with the absence of a varus or valgus thrust will improve the chance for successful knee ligament reconstruction.

VASCULAR ASSESSMENT

Arterial injury may occur with acute multiple ligament knee injuries and knee dislocations. These arterial injuries may present as complete arterial disruptions or occlusions, or as intimal flap tears that may cause delayed arterial occlusion. Bicruciate knee ligament injuries have the same incidence as tibiofemoral dislocations that present unreduced. Initial vascular evaluation of the acute multiple ligament injured dislocated knee includes physical examination for symmetry of pulses between the injured and noninjured lower extremities, and ankle brachial index (ABI) measurements. Abnormal or asymmetrical pulses or an ABI of less than 0.9 indicates the need for vascular consultation, advanced arterial imaging studies, and potential vascular surgical intervention.[1–6] Deep venous thrombosis (DVT) can occur with multiple ligament (dislocated) knee injuries in both the acute and chronic settings, and evaluation for DVT may be considered.

Up to 12% of popliteal arteries may have abnormal branching patterns, and this may be important for planning surgical reconstruction in the multiple ligament injured knee.[6–10] In addition, a certain number of multiple knee ligament injury patients will have had arterial repair or reconstruction. It is important to know about potential abnormal branching patterns of the popliteal artery, and the location of arterial reconstructions, to avoid injury to these structures during multiple knee ligament reconstruction surgical procedures.

PERONEAL NERVE INJURY

Peroneal nerve injuries can occur with multiple knee ligament injuries and knee dislocations and may influence the outcomes of multiple ligament knee reconstruction surgery. Treatment options for the nerve injury include nerve repair, nerve grafting, and direct nerve transfer. The author's preferred treatment includes peroneal nerve decompression at the time of the initial knee ligament surgery. When the nerve is in continuity, serial electromyograms are obtained. When no nerve recovery is demonstrated, posterior tibial tendon transfer is performed.[11]

INSTABILITY PATTERNS

Identifying the multiple planes of instability in multiple knee ligament injury patients is essential for successful treatment of these injuries. The posterior and anterior cruciate ligament disruptions will lead to increased posterior and anterior laxity at 90° and 30° of knee flexion. Recognition and correction of the medial and lateral side instability are the keys to successful posterior and anterior cruciate ligament surgery.

There are 3 different types of instability patterns that the author has observed in medial and lateral side knee injuries.[12–14] These are type A (axial rotation instability only), type B (axial rotation instability combined with varus and/or valgus laxity with a soft endpoint), and type C (axial rotation instability combined with varus and/or valgus laxity with little or no endpoint). The axial rotation instability (type A) medial or lateral side is most frequently overlooked. It is also critical to understand that combined medial and lateral side instability of different types occur with bicruciate and unicruciate multiple ligament knee injuries. Examples include posterior cruciate ligament, anterior cruciate ligament , lateral side type C, and medial side type A, or PCL, medial side type B, and lateral side type A instability patterns.

A combination of careful clinical examination, radiographs, and MRI studies aid in determining the correct diagnosis of multiple ligament knee injuries. Knee examination under anesthesia combined with fluoroscopy, stress radiography, and diagnostic arthroscopy also contributes to accurately diagnosing the multiple planes of instability.[15–17]

SURGICAL TIMING

Surgical timing in the multiple ligament injured (dislocated) knee is influenced by the vascular status of the injured extremity, the medial and lateral side injury severity, the postreduction stability, and additional surgical timing modifiers or considerations. Delayed reconstruction of 2 to 3 weeks may result in less postoperative motion loss. The author's ideal surgical approach is a single-stage procedure performed within 2 to 4 weeks of the patient's initial injury. Ideal surgical timing is not always possible. Surgical timing modifiers and considerations in the acute multiple ligament injured (dislocated) knee that may cause surgery to be performed earlier or later than what the surgeon considers ideal include vascular injuries, irreducible dislocations, open injuries, skin condition, extensor mechanism disruption, reduction stability, fractures or articular surface injuries, head trauma, and visceral injuries. The take-home message is that ideal surgical timing is not always possible, staged surgical reconstruction may be required, and the use of external fixation when acute stabilization is required until the definitive treatment can be performed. When staged reconstruction is used, the knee must be protected between stages so the initial stage reconstruction is not compromised with overaggressive physical activity.[18–22]

EXTERNAL FIXATION

External fixation is a useful tool in the management of the multiple ligament injured knee. Preoperative indications for the use of spanning external fixation include open dislocations, vascular repair, and inability to maintain reduction.[23] The advantages of using spanning external fixation include skin assessment, compartment pressure observation, and monitoring the neurovascular status of the affected limb. Preoperative use of external fixation compared with brace immobilization may lead to less terminal flexion postoperatively; however, this may be more dependent on injury severity of the involved extremity than the use of the spanning external fixation device.[21] Postoperative protection of multiple knee ligament reconstructions in a hinged external fixation device may lead to more favorable static stability than postoperative brace immobilization.[24] The use of spanning external fixation in treatment of the multiple ligament injured knee preoperatively and postoperatively is based on the individual case.

If the author can control the knee in a brace, he uses a brace. If he cannot control the knee in a brace, he uses an external fixation device. Postapplication radiogaphs are used to confirm initial reduction and to confirm that reduction is maintained. Occasionally, the author has used a spanning external fixator for treatment of the multiple ligament injured knee in patients who are not surgical candidates.

SUMMARY

- The multiple ligament injured knee (knee dislocation) is oftentimes part of a multisystem injury complex that can include injuries not only to knee ligaments but also to blood vessels, skin, nerves, bones (fractures), head, and other organ system trauma. These additional injuries can affect surgical timing for knee ligament reconstruction and also affect the results of treatment.
- Fracture reduction and fixation must be achieved to determine instability patterns, and intra-articular fractures must be reduced and stabilized to protect future ligament reconstructions.
- Lower-extremity malalignment with varus or valgus thrust during the stance phase of gait should be corrected with osteotomy before ligament reconstruction to maximize the chance for successful knee ligament reconstruction results.
- Arterial and venous assessment in the acute (and chronic) multiple ligament injured knee is important to evaluate for acute arterial injuries, DVT, abnormal popliteal artery branching patterns, and the location of arterial repair and reconstructions in the multiple ligament injured knee.
- Peroneal nerve injuries may occur in the multiple ligament injured (dislocated) knee and can be treated by peroneal nerve decompression, nerve repair, nerve grafting, direct nerve transfer, and tendon transfer. It is important to avoid heel cord contracture and equinus deformity at the foot and ankle because this will cause the knee to hyperextend during the stance phase of gait and may compromise knee ligament reconstruction.
- Correct diagnosis with recognition and correction of the medial and lateral side instability is the key to successful posterior and anterior cruciate ligament surgery.
- Surgical timing in the multiple ligament injured (dislocated) knee is influenced by the vascular status of the injured extremity, the medial and lateral side injury severity, the postreduction stability, and additional surgical timing modifiers or considerations. Ideal surgical timing is not always possible. Staged surgical reconstruction may be required, and external fixation may be used when acute stabilization is required until the definitive treatment can be performed.
- The use of spanning external fixation in treatment of the multiple ligament injured knee preoperatively and postoperatively is based on the individual case. If the author can control the knee in a brace, he uses a brace. If he cannot control the knee in a brace, he uses an external fixation device. Postapplication radiographs are used to confirm initial reduction and that reduction is maintained.

REFERENCES

1. Green NE, Allen BL. Vascular injuries associated with dislocation of the knee. J Bone Joint Surg Am 1977;59A:236–9.
2. Welling RE, Kakkasseril J, Cranley JJ. Complete dislocations of the knee with popliteal vascular injury. J Trauma 1981;21(6):450–3.
3. Wascher DC, Dvirnik PC, Decoster TA. Knee dislocation: initial assessment and implications for treatment. J Orthop Trauma 1997;11:525–9.

4. Kennedy JC. Complete dislocations of the knee joint. J Bone Joint Surg Am 1963; 45:889–904.
5. Mills WJ, Barei DP, McNair P. The value of the ankle-brachial index for diagnosing arterial injury after knee dislocation: a prospective study. J Trauma 2004;56(6): 1261–5.
6. Wascher DC. High-velocity knee dislocation with vascular injury. Treatment principles. Clin Sports Med 2000;19(3):457–77.
7. Mavili E, Donmez H, Kahriman G, et al. Popliteal artery branching patterns detected by digital subtraction angiography. Diagn Interv Radiol 2011;17:80–3.
8. Butt U, Samuel R, Sahu A, et al. Arterial injury in total knee arthroplasty. J Arthroplasty 2010;25(8):1311–8.
9. Kim D, Orron D, Skillman J. Surgical significance of popliteal artery variants. A unified angiographic classification. Ann Surg 1989;210(6):776–81.
10. Keser S, Savranlar A, Bavar A, et al. Anatomic localization of the popliteal artery at the level of the knee joint: a magnetic resonance imaging study. Arthroscopy 2006;22(6):656–9.
11. Cush G, Malony P, Irgit K. Drop foot after knee dislocation: evaluation and treatment. In: Fanelli GC, editor. The multiple ligament injured knee: a practical guide to management. 2nd edition. New York: Springer; 2013. p. 343–53.
12. Fanelli GC, Feldman DD. Management of combined anterior cruciate ligament/ posterior cruciate ligament/posterolateral complex injuries of the knee. Oper Tech Sports Med 1999;7(3):143–9.
13. Fanelli GC, Harris JD. Late MCL (medial collateral ligament) reconstruction. Techniques in Knee Surgery 2007;6(2):99–105.
14. Fanelli GC, Harris JD. Surgical treatment of acute medial collateral ligament and posteromedial corner injuries of the knee. Sports Med Arthrosc Rev 2006;14(2): 78–83.
15. Fanelli GC, Giannotti B, Edson CJ. Current concepts review. The posterior cruciate ligament: arthroscopic evaluation and treatment. Arthroscopy 1994;10(6): 673–88.
16. Fanelli GC. Arthroscopic evaluation of the PCL. In: Fanelli GC, editor. Posterior cruciate ligament injuries. A practical guide to management. New York: Springer-Verlag; 2001. p. 95–105.
17. LaPrade RF. Arthroscopic evaluation of the lateral compartment of knees with grade 3 posterolateral knee complex injuries. Am J Sports Med 1997;25(5): 596–602.
18. Fanelli GC, Orcutt DR, Edson CJ. The multiple-ligament injured knee: evaluation, treatment, and results. Arthroscopy 2005;21(4):471–86.
19. Mook WR, Miller MD, Diduch DR, et al. Multiple-ligament knee injuries: a systematic review of the timing of operative intervention and postoperative rehabilitation. J Bone Joint Surg Am 2009;91(12):2946–57.
20. Levy B, Dajani KA, Whalen DB, et al. Decision making in the multiple ligament injured knee: an evidence based systematic review. Arthroscopy 2009;25(4): 430–8.
21. Levy B, Fanelli GC, Whalen D, et al. Modern perspectives for the treatment of knee dislocations and multiligament reconstruction. J Am Acad Orthop Surg 2009;17(4):197–206.
22. Fanelli GC, Stannard JP, Stuart MJ, et al. Management of complex knee ligament injuries. J Bone Joint Surg Am 2010;92(12):2235–46.
23. Stuart MJ. Evaluation and treatment principles of knee dislocations. Oper Tech Sports Med 2001;9(2):91–5.

24. Stannard J, Nuelle C, McGwinn G, et al. Hinged external fixation in the treatment of knee dislocations: a prospective randomized study. J Bone Joint Surg Am 2014;96(3):184–91.

FURTHER READINGS

Fanelli GC, editor. The multiple ligament injured knee. A practical guide to management. 2nd edition. New York: Springer-Verlag; 2013.

Fanelli GC, editor. Posterior cruciate ligament injuries: a practical guide to management. 2nd edition. New York: Springer; 2015.

Vascular Injury in the Multiligament Injured Knee

Graeme Matthewson, MD[a],*, Adam Kwapisz, MD, PhD[a,b], Treny Sasyniuk, MSc[a],
Peter MacDonald, MD, FRCSC[a]

KEYWORDS

- Vasc injury • MLIK • Knee dislocation • Compartment syndrome • External fixation
- Bypass graft

KEY POINTS

- Vascular injury following a knee injury, although rare, is a potentially devastating injury that could result in loss of life or limb.
- Any suspected multiligament knee injury should undergo a thorough physical examination and an ankle-brachial index (ABI). If the ABI is <0.9, further assessment with advanced imaging to determine vascular status should occur.
- Prompt diagnosis and treatment of vascular injuries is key to avoiding complications such as amputation.
- Knee injuries in the obese population should have a high index of suspicion for atraumatic dislocation and should be examined for vascular injury due to the high rate of occurrence.

INTRODUCTION

A traumatic knee dislocation (KD), more commonly referred to as a "multiple ligament injured knee" (MLIK), is a rare event with an incidence estimated between 0.02% and 0.2% of all musculoskeletal injuries.[1] Because of the propensity for spontaneous reduction, it has been estimated that up to 50% of cases go unreported,[2] particularly in the polytrauma setting.[3–6] Although most MLIKs are thought to occur in the traumatic setting, there is an almost equal distribution that occurs through a low-velocity versus high-velocity mechanism (53% vs 47% respectively),[7] and 5% to 17% presenting as an open injury.[8]

The classification of KDs was first described by Kennedy in 1963.[9] Categories were based on the relative displacement of the tibia from the femur (anterior, posterior, medial, lateral, and rotatory dislocations). The Kennedy classification system did not, however, take into account damage to the soft tissues or any other significant

[a] Orthopaedic Surgery, Pan Am Clinic, University of Manitoba, 75 Poseidon Bay, Winnipeg, Manitoba R3M 3E4, Canada; [b] Clinic of Orthopedics and Pediatric Orthopedics, Medical University of Lodz, Pomorska 251, 92-213, Lodz, Poland
* Corresponding author.
E-mail address: graememathewson@icloud.com

Clin Sports Med 38 (2019) 199–213
https://doi.org/10.1016/j.csm.2018.11.001   **sportsmed.theclinics.com**
0278-5919/19/Crown Copyright © 2018 Published by Elsevier Inc. All rights reserved.

associated injuries. The most common classification system used today is by Schenck,[10] who designed a grading system that delineates the ligamentous injuries associated with the dislocation (**Fig. 1**).

Although the Schenck system takes into account the ligamentous damage, it fails to address neurovascular injuries. In a review of 303 patients with traumatic KD, Moatshe and colleagues[1] found that most cases involved 3 ligaments (52% KDIII-M and 28% KDIII-L) with 19% suffering a peroneal nerve injury (10.9% partial and 8.3% complete) and 5% a vascular injury. Contrary to the popular belief that KDIII-M injuries have the highest rate of vascular compromise, a meta-analysis performed by Medina and colleagues[11] found the highest rate of vascular injury was in KDIII-L knees (32%) followed by those with a posterior dislocation (25%). This finding was further supported by Moatshe and colleagues[1] and Sanders and colleagues,[12] with Moatshe and colleagues[1] observing a ninefold increased risk of vascular injury in the KDIII-L subtype. Because of the high-energy mechanism of traumatic MLIK injuries, clinicians should have a high index of suspicion for a vascular injury, particularly to the popliteal artery, as it has been reported in 12% to 80% of MLIK cases.[13–15] In a more recent study reviewing 8500 cases in North America, this statistic was reduced to only 3.3% of cases.[16]

In addition to high-energy injuries, risk factors that increase the likelihood of a vascular injury include obesity and open injuries, with a 7% and more than 300% increased risk, respectively.[17] Obesity is of particular concern,[18] as forces ranging from 2 to 4 times body weight are sustained during ambulation, which may exceed the threshold of the ligamentous structures. Dislocation could occur in seemingly benign and low-energy situations such as rising from a chair.[19] In their article on low-velocity KDs, Vaidya and colleagues[20] reported up to 27% of patients had a vascular injury and up to 10% of morbidly obese patients required surgical intervention.[21] Hagino and colleagues[22] reported on spontaneous KD in the morbidly obese population in which each case resulted in vascular compromise. With the increasing rate of obesity in North America, there should be a high index of suspicion for a vascular injury in this population, and every case should undergo a thorough neurovascular examination.

VASCULAR INJURY

Associated vascular compromise accompanying an MLIK is a potential life-threatening and limb-threatening complication.[7,23] Nearly 20% to 30% [24,25] of these injuries could result in limb amputation, increasing up to 80% with ischemic episodes lasting more than 8 hours from the time of injury.[24] In a series of 63 individuals, 30% of the individuals were operated on within 6 hours of injury without requiring

Schenck Classification	
KD I	Multiligamenous injury with ACL or PCL involvement (1 ligament)
KD II	ACL and PCL Injury (2 ligaments)
KD III	ACL + PCL + PMC or PLC (3 ligaments) M = ACL, PCL, MCL L = ACL, PCL, LCL
KD IV	Injury to ACL, PCL, PMC and PLC (4 ligaments)
KD V	Multiligamentous injury with periarticular fracture

Fig. 1. KD classification by Schenck and colleagues. PMC, posteromedial corner. (*From* Schenck R. Classification of knee dislocations. In: The multiple ligament injured knee: a practical guide to management. Springer Science & Business Media; 2004. p. 10; with permission.)

amputation.[25] Overall, the rate of vascular injury requiring surgical intervention has been estimated at 5.63%.[21] This estimate is based on a study by Johnson and colleagues[21] in which they reviewed 19,087 MLIKs. However, when identified, repair of the popliteal artery has been shown to decrease the rate of amputation by as much as 40%, from 73% down to 32% in those with vascular repair.[26]

MLIKs are particularly susceptible to vascular injuries due to several anatomic factors relating to their intimate relationship with surrounding tissues. Cadaveric studies describe the popliteal artery's tight adherence to the medial femoral epicondyle at the adductor hiatus (the distal extent of Hunters canal), as well as its fixation distally to the tendinous arch of the soleus. This vascular tether makes it quite vulnerable to any excessive anterior or posterior translations, including complete dislocation.[15,27,28] This relationship causes the popliteal vascular bundle to be prone to intima disruption, dissection, thrombosis, pseudo-aneurysm, and partial or even complete transection.[29] Due to this orientation, posterior dislocations tend to cause direct compression of the vessel and full-thickness tears, whereas anterior dislocations result in a traction injury causing partial-thickness defects in the vessel wall.[13]

Historically it was believed that an MLIK resulted in an arterial flow disturbance due to an intimal tear in the popliteal artery, which then progressed to thrombus formation and subsequent vessel occlusion at the site of damage. Therefore, an aggressive approach, with excision of the damaged segment, was recommended.[30] However, more recent studies have demonstrated that the progression from an intimal tear with no disruption of vascular flow, to complete occlusion is quite rare, leading many surgeons to observe patients found to have a normal initial neurovascular examination, and follow them with frequent serial examinations.[31]

DIAGNOSIS
Acute Setting

The missed diagnosis of a popliteal artery injury could be potentially disastrous for the management of an MLIK and therefore a thorough neurovascular assessment should be performed before any intervention or surgical management, particularly when considering the use of a tourniquet.[32] In a suspected MLIK, an expedited assessment is paramount, with the goal of any vascular injury to be identified within the first 8 hours from the time of injury to diminish the risk of requiring a subsequent limb amputation.[14,33]

Physical Examination and Imaging

Initially trauma practitioners relied solely on physical examination by checking a patient's distal pulses and occasionally performing an ankle-brachial index (ABI).[34] If any abnormalities were identified on physical examination, this was closely followed by angiography as the diagnostic modality of choice. However, this approach was deemed an inefficient use of resources and an unnecessary exposure to excess radiation, with newer reports suggesting a decision-making algorithm based on physical examination and the use of MRI or computed tomography (CT) imaging rather than angiography.[23,35–37] There are numerous protocols described in the literature with a few subtle variations. The differences lie mainly in the number of, and the time intervals in which, to perform serial examinations. Many studies also differ on the utilization of a Doppler examination or the performance of an ABI. Despite these discrepancies, the reliability of these algorithms in their ability to diagnose potential vascular complications seems to be quite high.[38–45]

Based on their clinical experience, Nicandri and colleagues[35] suggested a protocol in which a baseline physical examination and ABI are performed (**Fig. 2**). They suggest that with any ABI greater than 0.9 and the presence of a palpable distal pulse, that further diagnostic workup with an arteriogram may not be required.[35] ABI testing has proven to be a reliable and safe test with 95% to 100% sensitivity and 80% to 100% specificity in detecting surgically appropriate vascular injuries.[42] Unfortunately, in a retrospective review of 25 cases, Parker and colleagues[24] found that in 19 of 25 cases, the treating physicians relied solely on the warmth of the patient's feet without documenting the status of the distal pulses. In this cohort, only 2 patients had documented ABIs.[23] This practice ignores the recommendations made by Jones and colleagues[46] in 1979, when they reported that pulse testing alone is not sufficient in the diagnostic workup of vascular injuries. Their reasoning is mainly due to the ability of the collateral circulation to maintain peripheral pulses, even in the setting of a complete rupture of the popliteal artery.[14,46,47] For this reason, it has been suggested that pulse testing should be followed by an ABI with values lower than 0.9 being considered for further diagnostic testing.[37] In such cases, Nicandri and colleagues[35] recommend performing an arteriogram; however, in cases in which the distal pulses are completely absent, surgical exploration should be performed immediately. As with most practice, this approach is not considered universal, with some investigators suggesting an arteriogram or MR arthrography on all patients who have suffered a KD regardless of ABI findings.[48] In this setting, MR arteriography would have the advantage of being able to perform a conventional MRI to evaluate any concomitant ligamentous injuries while also assessing the vascular status.[28]

Although this protocol has been proven to be reliable, its utilization remains a challenge, with 1 article reporting that only 81% of MLIK cases were managed with a proper algorithm.[23,24,35,49] Maslaris and colleagues[49] also recommended an assessment protocol that includes ABI and peripheral pulse testing followed by CT angiography (CTA) if the patient has an abnormality on examination, or, if there is any restriction in clinical assessment. CTA itself has been described as a reliable, less invasive and therefore less dangerous imaging modality. However, some investigators prefer to use MRI angiography amid concerns of excess radiation exposure found with

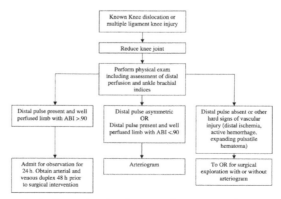

Fig. 2. Approach to physical examination in MLIK. (*From* Nicandri GT, Dunbar RP, Wahl CJ. Are evidence-based protocols which identify vascular injury associated with knee dislocation underutilized? Knee Surg Sports Traumat Arthrosc Off J ESSKA 2010;18:1005–12; with permission.)

CTA,[50–53] as well as the previously mentioned benefits of ligamentous evaluation. As MLIK is commonly complicated by Common Peroneal Nerve (CPN) injury in up to 45% of cases, Maslaris and colleagues[49] created a detailed protocol for MLIK management influenced by recent treatment algorithms published for vascular injury as well as the CPN assessment protocol described by Woodmass and colleagues.[49,54,55] This protocol describes in detail the possible scenarios as well as the suggested management for each outcome (**Fig. 3**).

TREATMENT
Reduction and Initial Immobilization

In each case, the treatment of an MLIK starts with immediate reduction and immobilization, and occasionally immediate surgical intervention.[49,53] Initial immobilization acts to preserve soft tissue integrity while maintaining the perfusion of the limb.[49] However, to date there is no agreed on method of immobilization determined in the literature. Commonly today, the use of an external fixator (ExFix) is more in favor as compared with casting or bracing. A few investigators have suggested that earlier range of motion may be beneficial in preserving cartilage and decreasing joint stiffness.[31,56–62] Therefore, a hinged ExFix has been advocated by some investigators, along with initial short-term immobilization, to allow preliminary stabilization of the soft tissues.[13,63] Maintenance of reduction aids in ameliorating the traction forces that occurs with a maligned knee joint, particularly to the posterior vasculature, due to the proximal and distal tethers.[64]

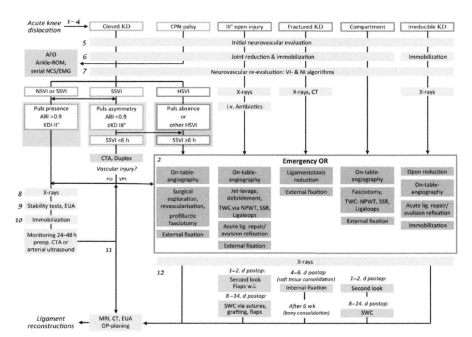

Fig. 3. Combined treatment pathway determined by the presence of concomitant injuries. (*From* Maslaris A, Brinkmann O, Bungartz M, et al. Management of knee dislocation prior to ligament reconstruction: what is the current evidence? Update of a universal treatment algorithm. Eur J Orthop Surg Traumatol 2018. https://doi.org/10.1007/s00590-018-2148-4; with permission.)

Ligamentous Stabilization and Vascular Repair

Following an initial period of immobilization, most surgeons would opt for further ligamentous reconstruction/repair, as surgical treatment has been shown to be superior to immobilization in the setting of high-energy KDs.[65,66] A similar approach should be applied to all patients suffering an MLIK; however, in some cases in which limb perfusion is compromised, immediate surgical intervention is necessary. In such cases, numerous treatment approaches have been reported.[12,49,53] In the event of a vascular injury, ligamentous repair should be performed in a delayed fashion following restoration of circulation to the distal extremity.[33]

Vascular injuries following an MLIK can be quite variable with a wide spectrum of treatment options ranging from observation to arterial bypass grafting.[15,67] Initial experiences from World War II revealed that popliteal artery ligation in the acute setting resulted in an amputation rate of nearly 70% or more in both military[68] and civilian populations.[69] This incidence decreased dramatically to fewer than 30% following the advent of surgical repair during the Vietnam[70] and Korean[71] wars. Once a significant popliteal artery injury is identified, revascularization with arterial repair for short segmental lesions and bypass grafting for more severely damaged areas may be indicated.[53]

Following repair, the limb should be maintained in reduction to protect the graft for 2 to 6 weeks depending on the status of the soft tissues before further surgical intervention. This can be performed as mentioned previously either through initial static immobilization (static ExFix) followed by hinged mobilization, or through the use of a hinged external fixator or hinged knee brace.[72] Even when vascular repair and stabilization is received within 8 hours from injury, the incidence of affected limb amputation may still reach as high as 30%.[23]

Compartment Syndrome

The development or presence of compartment syndrome (CS) should always be evaluated in the initial workup of an MLIK, as this will help dictate the initial steps in the surgical decision-making process. Early signs of CS include pain out of proportion that is particularly resistant to opioid analgesics, as well as pain with passive flexion/extension of the great toe or ankle. In less obvious cases in which a patient is obtunded or intubated and exhibits signs concerning for CS, such as unexplained tachycardia and tense lower extremity compartments, then compartment pressures should be measured. It is widely reported that pressures exceeding an absolute value of 30 mm Hg in a hemodynamically stable patient and a pressure measuring less than 30 mm Hg delta pressure (difference between diastolic blood pressure and compartment pressure measurement) in a hemodynamically unstable patient, are appropriate indications for urgent fasciotomy. Continuous observations with minimal intervals are suggested when symptoms and pressures are regarded as borderline.[73–75] In the setting of a vascular injury, the development of a CS begins with the primary period of ischemia, exacerbated by a secondary injury following vascular reperfusion.[76] This secondary injury is thought to arise from free radical release in addition to the local inflammatory response initiated by the breakdown of tissues and their degradation products, as a consequence of the ischemic episode.[77] This results in increased tissue edema and followed by an increase in compartmental pressures. In the trauma setting, this may be compounded by fracture and hematoma formation as well.[78] In the setting of prolonged warm ischemia time (4–6 hours), many investigators recommend performing a prophylactic fasciotomy regardless of the symptomatology.[53,56,78] Other indications for fasciotomy in lieu of the classic physical findings include a multiply injured extremity (fracture and vascular injury) as well as for prophylaxis before aeromedical transport where proper monitoring and the ability to perform a fasciotomy are limited.[78] With regard to exposure, in the vascular setting there is no rationale to perform a limited fasciotomy, as the consequences of an incomplete release in this setting could result in limb amputation or even death.[79]

Prognosis

Following an MLIK, patients notice a considerable difference in the function of their injured knee. Some reports show satisfaction ratings as high as 80%,[80] whereas others report good to excellent results in only 33% with residual symptoms in up to 86% of cases.[8] Most series, however, show that many patients suffer from serious disability after even an isolated ligamentous injury alone,[65] with a return to work rate of only 54% in an active military population.[81] In the setting of a vascular injury, results are further diminished. First addressed by Patterson and colleagues[33] as part of the Lower Extremity Assessment Project (LEAP) study in 2007, those who suffered a limb-threatening KD had moderate to high levels of disability at 2 years and close to 20% of patients presenting to hospital with limb ischemia required an amputation.

Following this, Sanders and colleagues[12] reported in 2017 that MLIKs with vascular involvement treated with bypass graft sustained worse functional outcome scores when compared with the rest of MLIK patients. They found the mean International Knee Documentation Committee (IKDC) and Lysholm scores for patients with a vascular injury were 59.7 and 62.5 as compared with 83.8 and 86.4 in those with only a ligamentous injury, respectively. In their cohort, most injuries were KDLIII (29/48), which was represented evenly in the vascular (10/16) and control groups (19/32). However, it should be noted, that currently there are no clinically validated outcome scores specifically for the MLIK,[82] with considerable discrepancy in functional outcome scores between the IKDC and Lysholm scores.[83]

CASE EXAMPLE

A 19-year-old man presented to a northern remote nursing station following a hyperextension injury to his right knee while running down a hill. He was taken to the nursing station because of concerns of a decreased pulse in his leg and an obvious deformity to his knee. ABIs performed at that time came back as 0.54. A reduction was attempted before transport; however, it was unsuccessful and the patient was rapidly transported to our institution. During transport, the patient reported increasing pain to the right leg that was not responsive to narcotics. The patient arrived with the knee still dislocated and the foot stuck in equinus. The operating room (OR) was booked for an emergency surgery and a repeat attempt at a closed reduction was unsuccessful. CTA revealed a persistently posteriorly dislocated tibia with complete occlusion of the popliteal artery (**Fig. 4**). At the time of the OR, the time from injury had reached 9 hours and the compartments of the leg were very tense. The decision to perform a 4-compartment fasciotomy was made. Following fasciotomy, the muscle was very dark in appearance. A 4-pin external fixator construct was placed (**Fig. 5**); however, the knee was not completely reducible, as a suspected torn lateral meniscus was preventing complete reduction. A vascular surgeon then isolated and dissected out the popliteal artery, which was thrombosed with a large hematoma tracking down the deep posterior compartment. They gave 7000 units of intravenous heparin and performed a reversed saphenous vein graft achieving excellent pulsatile flow to the distal popliteal artery (**Fig. 6**). Because of the position of the vein graft and swelling, closure of the fasciotomy sites was not performed at that time. Six days later, the patient was

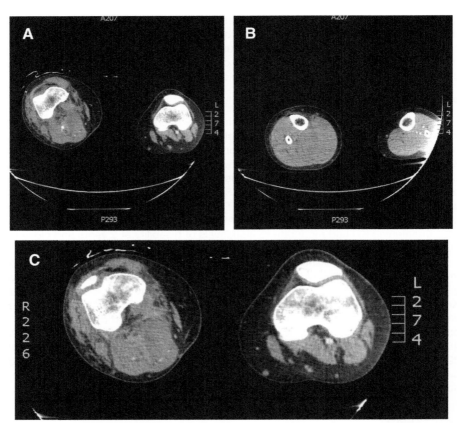

Fig. 4. CT angiogram. (*A*) Popliteal artery proximal to occlusion. (*B*) Popliteal artery distal to occlusion, midway down leg. (*C*) Popliteal artery at the level of the occlusion.

taken for debridement and closure of the fasciotomy sites. The muscle appeared pink and bleeding; however, there was still minimal contraction at this point in time. Still unable to perform a primary closure because of wound size and tension over the graft site, several split-thickness skin grafts were harvested from the contralateral thigh and were meshed and stapled in place over the fasciotomy sites. Mepitel silicone sheaths were placed on top and Xeroform to apply pressure in order for the grafts to conform to the wound. Postoperatively, the patient was sent for an MRI to assess the damaged structures of the knee. The MRI showed injury to all 4 ligaments of the knee (anterior cruciate [ACL], posterior cruciate [PCL], medial collateral [MCL], and lateral collateral ligaments [LCL]), as well as the lateral and medial menisci. Two weeks later, after healing of the graft sites, the patient was taken back to the OR for ligament reconstruction. At that time, it was found that the patient had a rupture of the ACL and PCL, LCL and MCL rupture, lateral meniscus bucket handle tear, injury to the popliteus and biceps femoris (posterolateral corner injury), as well as an injury to the semimembranosus tendon. In order of surgical procedure, a diagnostic scope was performed identifying the damaged structures followed by debridement of any loose flaps on the chondral surfaces of the distal femur and lateral plateau. A medial horn tear was then identified and debrided back to a stable base, which was unfortunately deemed

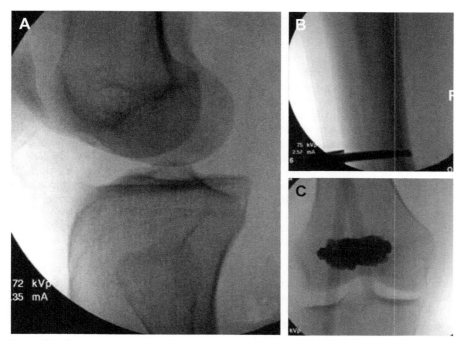

Fig. 5. (*A*) Fluoroscopic image after attempted reduction with ExFix with slight posterior subluxation due to entrapped meniscus. (*B*) Lateral image of the tibial pin. (*C*) AP image of the femoral pin showing widening of the lateral compartment.

irreparable. The lateral meniscus was identified and found to be dislocated out the back of the knee, preventing the tibia from reducing anteriorly and was unable to be reduced arthroscopically. A PCL drill guide was used to drill an 11-mm tunnel at the isometric point of the femur, followed by passing of an Achilles tendon allograft with

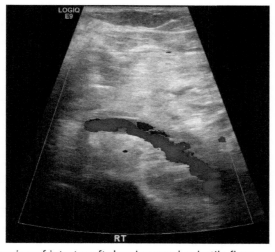

Fig. 6. Doppler imaging of intact graft showing good pulsatile flow.

bone block. The lateral side of the knee was then addressed with a lateral approach and the popliteus, biceps femoris, and LCL ruptures were identified with difficulty, as the soft tissues had already begun to heal since the time of injury. The peroneal nerve was then dissected out over a 12-cm distance with a focal 3-cm hemorrhagic section identified and scarring around the nerve. Through the lateral incision, the lateral meniscus was brought back inside the knee and the knee was reduced. The lateral meniscus was then arthroscopically repaired with 3 inside meniscal sutures that were later tied down at the end of the case. Attention was then shifted to the medial side of the knee. A medial incision was performed, remaining just in the margins of the fasciotomy wounds. The superficial MCL and semimembranosus were peeled off the femur in a sleeve up to the femoral epicondyle and the capsule was released off the back of the femur, being careful not to disrupt the vascular graft. A trough was made in the posterior tibia and the Achilles tendon graft with bone block was passed through the knee and arthroscopically passed into the tunnel created in the medial femoral condyle. The lateral structures were then secured to the fibular head using 2 anchors, as well as 1 anchor in the sulcus for the popliteus repair. A tunnel was created in the fibular head and a semitendinosus allograft was passed through and secured through a tunnel at the isometric point on the femur. The medial site structures were repaired using 2 suture anchors secured to the tibia that were tied at the end of the case under appropriate tension. The PCL was then secured to the femur using an interference screw, as the tibial side had already been secured using a 4.5-mm cannulated screw. The LCL reconstruction was then secured in place with the knee in 30° of flexion and slight valgus force applied. The repairs were then sequentially tied down starting with the biceps femoris, popliteus, and then the LCL repair, followed by the superficial MCL and semimembranosus repair. This resulted in a stable knee on testing that was well reduced on fluoroscopic imaging (**Fig. 7**). Having stabilized

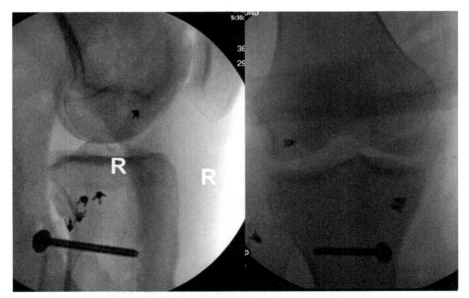

Fig. 7. Fluoroscopic image showing reduced knee with final implants in position. Lateral (*left*) and AP (*right*) images of a concentrically reduced knee post ligamentous reconstruction.

the knee, attention was then shifted to the equinus contracture of the right ankle and a tendon-Achilles-lengthening was performed. The plan for ACL reconstruction was to come back once the patient had achieved near-normal range of motion. It was this surgeon's preferred method to reconstruct the ACL in a young or athletic patient population once they had regained close to normal range of motion of the knee and to reconstruct older populations only if they later became symptomatic.

SUMMARY

The MLIK, although rare, is a devastating injury with the potential for loss of life and limb due to susceptibility of an associated vascular injury. Dislocations of the knee can occur through low-energy and high-energy mechanisms and do so at almost equal rates. Clinicians should be aware of the potential for a spontaneous dislocation in the morbidly obese and have a high index of suspicion for vascular injury in this population. Proper management of the MLIK requires prompt diagnosis, immediate reduction, and a thorough assessment of the vascular status of the limb. Diagnosis should be initiated with a thorough physical examination, followed by vascular studies, such as an ABI, CT, MR or traditional angiogram. If vascular damage warrants surgery, then ligamentous repair should be delayed until circulation to the distal extremity has been restored and soft tissue swelling permits. When an MLIK involves both the ACL and PCL, the reconstructions can be staged or performed in the same setting. Outcomes following an MLIK are modest and further diminished when associated with a significant vascular injury requiring repair, reconstruction, or amputation.

REFERENCES

1. Moatshe G, Dornan GJ, Løken S, et al. Demographics and injuries associated with knee dislocation: a prospective review of 303 patients. Orthop J Sports Med 2017;5(5). 2325967711770652.
2. Kapur S, Wissman RD, Robertson M, et al. Acute knee dislocation: review of an elusive entity. Curr Probl Diagn Radiol 2009;38(6):237–50.
3. Peskun CJ, Levy BA, Fanelli GC, et al. Diagnosis and management of knee dislocations. Phys Sportsmed 2010;38(4):101–11.
4. Howells NR, Brunton LR, Robinson J, et al. Acute knee dislocation: an evidence based approach to the management of the multiligament injured knee. Injury 2011;42(11):1198–204.
5. Hegyes MS, Richardson MW, Miller MD. Knee dislocation. Complications of nonoperative and operative management. Clin Sports Med 2000;19(3):519–43.
6. Cole BJ, Harner CD. The multiple ligament injured knee. Clin Sports Med 1999; 18(1):241–62.
7. Georgiadis AG, Mohammad FH, Mizerik KT, et al. Changing presentation of knee dislocation and vascular injury from high-energy trauma to low-energy falls in the morbidly obese. J Vasc Surg 2013;57(5):1196–203.
8. King JJ, Cerynik DL, Blair JA, et al. Surgical outcomes after traumatic open knee dislocation. Knee Surg Sports Traumatol Arthrosc 2009;17(9):1027–32.
9. Kennedy JC. Complete dislocation of the knee joint. J Bone Joint Surg Am 1963; 45:889–904.
10. Schenck R. Classification of knee dislocations. In: The multiple ligament injured knee: a practical guide to management. Springer Science & Business Media; 2004. p. 10.
11. Medina O, Arom GA, Yeranosian MG, et al. Vascular and nerve injury after knee dislocation: a systematic review. Clin Orthop 2014;472(9):2621–9.

12. Sanders TL, Johnson NR, Levy NM, et al. Effect of vascular injury on functional outcome in knees with multi-ligament injury: a matched-cohort analysis. J Bone Joint Surg Am 2017;99(18):1565–71.

13. Levy NM, Krych AJ, Hevesi M, et al. Does age predict outcome after multiligament knee reconstruction for the dislocated knee? 2- to 22-year follow-up. Knee Surg Sports Traumatol Arthrosc 2015;23(10):3003–7.

14. Green NE, Allen BL. Vascular injuries associated with dislocation of the knee. J Bone Joint Surg Am 1977;59(2):236.

15. McDonough EB, Wojtys EM. Multiligamentous injuries of the knee and associated vascular injuries. Am J Sports Med 2009;37(1):156–9.

16. Natsuhara KM, Yeranosian MG, Cohen JR, et al. What is the frequency of vascular injury after knee dislocation? Clin Orthop 2014;472(9):2615–20.

17. Weinberg DS, Scarcella NR, Napora JK, et al. Can vascular injury be appropriately assessed with physical examination after knee dislocation? Clin Orthop 2016;474(6):1453–8.

18. Henrichs A. A review of knee dislocations. J Athl Train 2004;39(4):365–9.

19. Marin EL, Bifulco SS, Fast A. Obesity. A risk factor for knee dislocation. Am J Phys Med Rehabil 1990;69(3):132–4.

20. Vaidya R, Roth M, Nanavati D, et al. Low-velocity knee dislocations in obese and morbidly obese patients. Orthop J Sports Med 2015;3(4). 2325967115575719.

21. Johnson JP, Kleiner J, Klinge SA, et al. Increased incidence of vascular injury in obese patients with knee dislocations. J Orthop Trauma 2018;32(2):82–7.

22. Hagino RT, DeCaprio JD, Valentine RJ, et al. Spontaneous popliteal vascular injury in the morbidly obese. J Vasc Surg 1998;28(3):458–62 [discussion: 462–3].

23. Nicandri GT, Chamberlain AM, Wahl CJ. Practical management of knee dislocations: a selective angiography protocol to detect limb-threatening vascular injuries. Clin J Sport Med 2009;19(2):125–9.

24. Parker S, Handa A, Deakin M, et al. Knee dislocation and vascular injury: 4 year experience at a UK Major Trauma Centre and vascular hub. Injury 2016;47(3):752–6.

25. Downs AR, MacDonald P. Popliteal artery injuries: civilian experience with sixty-three patients during a twenty-four year period (1960 through 1984). J Vasc Surg 1986;4(1):55–62.

26. Gable DR, Allen JW, Richardson JD. Blunt popliteal artery injury: is physical examination alone enough for evaluation? J Trauma 1997;43(3):541–4.

27. Dwyer T, Whelan D. Anatomical considerations in multiligament knee injury and surgery. J Knee Surg 2012;25(4):263–74.

28. Johnson ME, Foster L, DeLee JC. Neurologic and vascular injuries associated with knee ligament injuries. Am J Sports Med 2008;36(12):2448–62.

29. Karkos CD, Koudounas G, Giagtzidis IT, et al. Traumatic knee dislocation and popliteal artery injury: a case series. Ann Vasc Surg 2018. https://doi.org/10.1016/j.avsg.2018.01.084.

30. Wascher DC. High-velocity knee dislocation with vascular injury. Treatment principles. Clin Sports Med 2000;19(3):457–77.

31. Levy BA, Fanelli GC, Whelan DB, et al. Controversies in the treatment of knee dislocations and multiligament reconstruction. J Am Acad Orthop Surg 2009;17(4):197–206.

32. Marom N, Ruzbarsky JJ, Roselaar N, et al. Knee MLI injuries: common problems and solutions. Clin Sports Med 2018;37(2):281–91.

33. Patterson BM, Agel J, Swiontkowski MF, et al, LEAP Study Group. Knee disloca-
    tions with vascular injury: outcomes in the Lower Extremity Assessment Project
    (LEAP) Study. J Trauma 2007;63(4):855–8.
34. Sisto DJ, Warren RF. Complete knee dislocation. A follow-up study of operative
    treatment. Clin Orthop 1985;198:94–101.
35. Nicandri GT, Dunbar RP, Wahl CJ. Are evidence-based protocols which identify
    vascular injury associated with knee dislocation underutilized? Knee Surg Sports
    Traumatol Arthrosc 2010;18(8):1005–12.
36. McKee L, Ibrahim MS, Lawrence T, et al. Current concepts in acute knee disloca-
    tion: the missed diagnosis? Open Orthop J 2014;8:162–7.
37. Mills WJ, Barei DP, McNair P. The value of the ankle-brachial index for diagnosing
    arterial injury after knee dislocation: a prospective study. J Trauma 2004;56(6):
    1261–5.
38. Abou-Sayed H, Berger DL. Blunt lower-extremity trauma and popliteal artery in-
    juries: revisiting the case for selective arteriography. Arch Surg 2002;137(5):
    585–9.
39. Atteberry LR, Dennis JW, Russo-Alesi F, et al. Changing patterns of arterial in-
    juries associated with fractures and dislocations. J Am Coll Surg 1996;183(4):
    377–83.
40. Dennis JW, Menawat S, Von Thron J, et al. Efficacy of deep venous thrombosis
    prophylaxis in trauma patients and identification of high-risk groups. J Trauma
    1993;35(1):132–8 [discussion: 138–9].
41. Kendall RW, Taylor DC, Salvian AJ, et al. The role of arteriography in assessing
    vascular injuries associated with dislocations of the knee. J Trauma 1993;35(6):
    875–8.
42. Martinez D, Sweatman K, Thompson EC. Popliteal artery injury associated with
    knee dislocations. Am Surg 2001;67(2):165–7.
43. Miranda FE, Dennis JW, Veldenz HC, et al. Confirmation of the safety and accu-
    racy of physical examination in the evaluation of knee dislocation for injury of the
    popliteal artery: a prospective study. J Trauma 2002;52(2):247–51 [discussion:
    251–2].
44. Stannard JP, Sheils TM, Lopez-Ben RR, et al. Vascular injuries in knee disloca-
    tions: the role of physical examination in determining the need for arteriography.
    J Bone Joint Surg Am 2004;86-A(5):910–5.
45. Treiman GS, Yellin AE, Weaver FA, et al. Examination of the patient with a knee
    dislocation. The case for selective arteriography. Arch Surg 1992;127(9):
    1056–62 [discussion: 1062–3].
46. Jones RE, Smith EC, Bone GE. Vascular and orthopedic complications of knee
    dislocation. Surg Gynecol Obstet 1979;149(4):554–8.
47. Alberty RE, Goodfried G, Boyden AM. Popliteal artery injury with fractural dislo-
    cation of the knee. Am J Surg 1981;142(1):36–40.
48. Boisrenoult P, Lustig S, Bonneviale P, et al. Vascular lesions associated with bicru-
    ciate and knee dislocation ligamentous injury. Orthop Traumatol Surg Res 2009;
    95(8):621–6.
49. Maslaris A, Brinkmann O, Bungartz M, et al. Management of knee dislocation
    prior to ligament reconstruction: What is the current evidence? Update of a uni-
    versal treatment algorithm. Eur J Orthop Surg Traumatol 2018. https://doi.org/
    10.1007/s00590-018-2148-4.
50. Fanelli GC, Stannard JP, Stuart MJ, et al. Management of complex knee ligament
    injuries. J Bone Joint Surg Am 2010;92(12):2235–46.

51. Redmond JM, Levy BA, Dajani KA, et al. Detecting vascular injury in lower-extremity orthopedic trauma: the role of CT angiography. Orthopedics 2008; 31(8):761–7.
52. Potter HG, Weinstein M, Allen AA, et al. Magnetic resonance imaging of the multiple-ligament injured knee. J Orthop Trauma 2002;16(5):330–9.
53. Pardiwala DN, Rao NN, Anand K, et al. Knee dislocations in sports injuries. Indian J Orthop 2017;51(5):552–62.
54. Feliciano DV, Moore EE, West MA, et al. Western Trauma Association critical decisions in trauma: evaluation and management of peripheral vascular injury, part II. J Trauma Acute Care Surg 2013;75(3):391–7.
55. Woodmass JM, Romatowski NPJ, Esposito JG, et al. A systematic review of peroneal nerve palsy and recovery following traumatic knee dislocation. Knee Surg Sports Traumatol Arthrosc 2015;23(10):2992–3002.
56. Stuart MJ. Evaluation and treatment principles of knee dislocations. Oper Tech Sports Med 2001;9(2):91–5.
57. Angelini FJ, Helito CP, Bonadio MB, et al. External fixator for treatment of the subacute and chronic multi-ligament-injured knee. Knee Surg Sports Traumatol Arthrosc 2015;23(10):3012–8.
58. Stannard JP, Nuelle CW, McGwin G, et al. Hinged external fixation in the treatment of knee dislocations: a prospective randomized study. J Bone Joint Surg Am 2014;96(3):184–91.
59. Ibrahim SAR, Ahmad FHF, Salah M, et al. Surgical management of traumatic knee dislocation. Arthroscopy 2008;24(2):178–87.
60. Engebretsen L, Risberg MA, Robertson B, et al. Outcome after knee dislocations: a 2-9 years follow-up of 85 consecutive patients. Knee Surg Sports Traumatol Arthrosc 2009;17(9):1013–26.
61. Behrens F, Kraft EL, Oegema TR. Biochemical changes in articular cartilage after joint immobilization by casting or external fixation. J Orthop Res 1989;7(3): 335–43.
62. Ghosh P, Taylor TK, Pettit GD, et al. Effect of postoperative immobilisation on the regrowth of the knee joint semilunar cartilage: an experimental study. J Orthop Res 1983;1(2):153–64.
63. Levy BA, Dajani KA, Whelan DB, et al. Decision making in the multiligament-injured knee: an evidence-based systematic review. Arthroscopy 2009;25(4): 430–8.
64. Klineberg EO, Crites BM, Flinn WR, et al. The role of arteriography in assessing popliteal artery injury in knee dislocations. J Trauma 2004;56(4):786–90.
65. Dedmond BT, Almekinders LC. Operative versus nonoperative treatment of knee dislocations: a meta-analysis. Am J Knee Surg 2001;14(1):33–8.
66. Wong C-H, Tan J-L, Chang H-C, et al. Knee dislocations—a retrospective study comparing operative versus closed immobilization treatment outcomes. Knee Surg Sports Traumatol Arthrosc 2004;12(6):540–4.
67. Sillanpää PJ, Kannus P, Niemi ST, et al. Incidence of knee dislocation and concomitant vascular injury requiring surgery: a nationwide study. J Trauma Acute Care Surg 2014;76(3):715–9.
68. DeBakey ME, Simeone FA. Battle injuries of the arteries in World War II; an analysis of 2,471 cases. Ann Surg 1946;123:534–79.
69. Fabian TC, Turkleson ML, Connelly TL, et al. Injury to the popliteal artery. Am J Surg 1982;143(2):225–8.
70. Rich NM, Baugh JH, Hughes CW. Popliteal artery injuries in Vietnam. Am J Surg 1969;118(4):531–4.

71. Hughes CW. Arterial repair during the Korean war. Ann Surg 1958;147(4):555–61.
72. Moatshe G, Chahla J, LaPrade RF, et al. Diagnosis and treatment of multiligament knee injury: state of the art. J ISAKOS Jt Disord Orthop Sports Med 2017. https://doi.org/10.1136/jisakos-2016-000072.
73. Kakar S, Firoozabadi R, McKean J, et al. Diastolic blood pressure in patients with tibia fractures under anaesthesia: implications for the diagnosis of compartment syndrome. J Orthop Trauma 2007;21(2):99–103.
74. Mubarak SJ, Owen CA, Hargens AR, et al. Acute compartment syndromes: diagnosis and treatment with the aid of the wick catheter. J Bone Joint Surg Am 1978; 60(8):1091–5.
75. Matsen FA, Winquist RA, Krugmire RB. Diagnosis and management of compartmental syndromes. J Bone Joint Surg Am 1980;62(2):286–91.
76. Blebea J, Kerr JC, Shumko JZ, et al. Quantitative histochemical evaluation of skeletal muscle ischemia and reperfusion injury. J Surg Res 1987;43(4):311–21.
77. Ricci MA, Graham AM, Corbisiero R, et al. Are free radical scavengers beneficial in the treatment of compartment syndrome after acute arterial ischemia? J Vasc Surg 1989;9(2):244–50.
78. Percival TJ, White JM, Ricci MA. Compartment syndrome in the setting of vascular injury. Perspect Vasc Surg Endovasc Ther 2011;23(2):119–24.
79. Ganie FA, Lone H, Wani ML, et al. Role of liberal primary fasciotomy in traumatic vascular injury. Trauma Mon 2012;17(2):287–90.
80. Eranki V, Begg C, Wallace B. Outcomes of operatively treated acute knee dislocations. Open Orthop J 2010;4:22–30.
81. Ross AE, Taylor KF, Kirk KL, et al. Functional outcome of multiligamentous knee injuries treated arthroscopically in active duty soldiers. Mil Med 2009;174(10): 1133–7.
82. Dwyer T, Marx RG, Whelan D. Outcomes of treatment of multiple ligament knee injuries. J Knee Surg 2012;25(4):317–26.
83. Mariani PP, Santoriello P, Iannone S, et al. Comparison of surgical treatments for knee dislocation. Am J Knee Surg 1999;12(4):214–21.

The Biomechanics of Multiligament Knee Injuries
From Trauma to Treatment

Nicholas A. Trasolini, MD*, Adam Lindsay, MD,
Aaron Gipsman, MD, George F. Rick Hatch, MD

KEYWORDS

- Multiligamentous knee injury • Biomechanics • Knee dislocation • Internal bracing
- Ligament • Anterior cruciate • Posterior cruciate • Medial collateral

KEY POINTS

- The knee is comprised of primary and secondary stabilizers, all of which are critical to normal knee kinematics.
- Multiligamentous knee injuries are typically classified pathoanatomically, directionally, or by the ligaments involved.
- In the event of a knee dislocation with multiligamentous knee injury, it is important to recognize that total biomechanical disruption of the knee joint is greater than the sum of its individual ligamentous injuries.
- Limited biomechanical data exist for reconstructive options of the primary stabilizers of the knee in the context of multiligamentous knee injury.

INTRODUCTION

The knee joint is not a simple hinge. It is a complex organ with multiple layers of three-dimensional biomechanical constraints that endure high forces to sustain normal kinematics with 6° of freedom. The stability of the knee relies on a delicate balance of both primary and secondary restraints for coronal, sagittal, and rotational stability. Failure of these structures results in painful loss of function that can predispose patients to secondary soft tissue injuries or arthritis. Consequently, knee dislocations with multiple ligament injuries have severe biomechanical implications.

The objectives of this article are:

1. To review the biomechanics and kinematics of the knee joint
2. To outline the contributions of each primary and secondary knee stabilizer
3. To define the implications of multiligamentous knee injury (MLKI) patterns

Department of Orthopaedic Surgery, Keck Medical Center of the University of Southern California, 1520 San Pablo Street, Suite 2000, Los Angeles, CA 90033, USA
* Corresponding author.
E-mail address: nicholas.trasolinl@med.usc.edu

Clin Sports Med 38 (2019) 215–234
https://doi.org/10.1016/j.csm.2018.11.009
0278-5919/19/© 2018 Elsevier Inc. All rights reserved.

4. To summarize the biomechanical evidence for multiligamentous reconstruction techniques

KNEE STABILITY

Both primary and secondary stabilizers maintain knee stability in the sagittal, coronal, and axial planes. It is important in the context of multiple ligament injuries to understand both primary and secondary structures because secondary structures have an increased role in the presence of primary ligamentous injuries.

- The knee has 6° of freedom. These degrees of freedom are described in terms of 3 axes, each with 2 planes of motion.[1,2] The first axis is the tibial shaft axis, which defines internal and external tibial rotation, as well as proximal-distal translation. The second axis is the femoral epicondylar axis, which defines flexion and extension, as well as medial and lateral translation. The third is the anteroposterior axis, which is orthogonal to the other two. This axis determines the varus-valgus rotation and anterior-posterior translation.
- Stability in each plane is summarized in **Table 1**.

Rotational Stability

- Rotational knee stability is achieved by interplay between medial and lateral ligamentous constraints. The primary restraint to internal rotation in knee extension is the posterior oblique ligament (POL); in flexion, the primary restraint to internal rotation is the superficial medial collateral ligament (MCL).[3] Secondary restraints include the anterolateral ligament, posteromedial capsule (PMC), and anterior cruciate ligament (ACL).[3–5] The iliotibial band also resists internal rotation due to its anterolateral tibial attachment.[6] The primary restraints to external rotation are the posterolateral corner structures (PLC), including the lateral (fibular) collateral ligament (LCL), popliteofibular ligament (PFL), and popliteus.[3,7,8]

Coronal Stability

- Coronal knee stability is also controlled primarily by extra-articular structures. The primary restraint to valgus is the superficial MCL (sMCL), which is under

Table 1
Primary and secondary stabilizers in the knee

Plane	Motion	Primary Restraint	Secondary Restraints
Sagittal	Anterior translation	ACL	ALL,[86,87] menisci,[88,89] ITB,[86,87] MCL,[16] capsule, meniscocapsular, meniscotibial,[90] and meniscofemoral[91] attachments
	Posterior translation	PCL	MCL,[16] PLC, POL/PMC,[92] LCL, meniscofemoral ligaments[93]
Coronal	Varus	LCL	PFL,[94] popliteus[95]
	Valgus	Superficial MCL[96,97]	Deep MCL, POL, PMC[97]
Axial	Internal rotation	sMCL (in flexion)[3,98] POL (in extension)[3,98]	ACL,[98] ALL,[86] LCL,[77] PFL,[78] ITB(Kaplan fibers)[86]
	External rotation	LCL/PLC[95]	Popliteus,[95] PFL[94]

Abbreviations: ACL, anterior cruciate ligament; ALL, anterolateral ligament; ITB, iliotibial band; LCL, lateral collateral ligament; MCL, medial collateral ligament; PCL, posterior cruciate ligament; PFL, popliteofibular ligament; PLC, posterolateral corner; PMC, posteromedial capsule; POL, posterior oblique ligament; sMCL, superficial medial collateral ligament.

the most tension at 30° of knee flexion.[3] The secondary stabilizers to valgus include the deep MCL and ACL.[3] The primary stabilizer to varus is the LCL, with secondary contributions from the PLC structures.[3,8–10]

Sagittal Stability

- Sagittal knee stability is maintained by the intra-articular cruciate ligaments. The primary restraint against anterior tibial translation is the ACL.[3,11–13] Secondary restraints include the iliotibial band, PMC, anterolateral ligament, and menisci. There are also small secondary contributions from the MCL and LCL. The primary restraint against posterior tibial translation is the posterior cruciate ligament (PCL).[3,14,15] Secondary contributions come from the PLC, MCL, PMC and LCL.[3,16]

A detailed breakdown of the contributors to knee stability is outlined in **Tables 2–4**. This is organized by intra-articular, extra-articular, and articular components of knee stability. Intra-articular structures include the cruciate ligaments and menisci. Extra-articular structures include the collateral ligaments, PLC, and capsular ligaments (anterolateral ligament, POL, and PMC). Finally, the articular structures include the tibial slope, coronal alignment of the knee, lateral femoral condyle ratio, and medial femoral condyle sphericity.

In the context of multiple ligament injuries, secondary roles become increasingly important. For example, the MCL is not often considered a stabilizer against posterior tibial translation. However, in the case of of PCL deficiency, MCL sectioning increases posterior tibial translation by 350%.[3,16] Similarly, high-grade injuries to the PLC have been shown to increase forces within ACL reconstruction grafts.[17] In a cadaveric biomechanical model, partial and complete MCL injuries have been demonstrated to increase the anterior load and stress on the native ACL.[18]

Failure to address all factors contributing to instability can result in early failures or persistent instability. It is because of these relationships that many surgeons recommend treatment of all ligaments with $\geq$ grade 2 laxity and performing two-stage procedures when boney contributors to instability (eg, coronal malalignment) are present.[19]

INJURY BIOMECHANICS

The MLKI is a complex biomechanical problem that often results from a knee dislocation.[20] Knee dislocations are generally understood as ligamentous disruption with loss of tibiofemoral articular continuity, involving a combination of tears of the ACL, PCL, MCL, LCL, menisci, tendinous, and other stabilizing structures.[21] Ligamentous injury can be described by injury mechanisms and subsequently built into classifications.

Pathomechanics

- In their pathophysiologic approach to classification, Boisgard and colleagues[22] simplify the injury mechanisms down to gapping causing ligament tear, translation causing detachment, and rotation. These may occur in isolation, or in association, with isolated simple mechanisms being low energy, and combined mechanisms resulting from high-energy mechanisms.
- Simple gaping in a plane around a perpendicular axis, causes an initial peripheral ligament injury of the convex structure with subsequent cruciate ligament injury. Valgus loads cause medial lesions, varus loads cause lateral lesions, and hyperextension loads cause posterior lesions.

Table 2
Intra-articular components of stability include the ACL, PCL, and menisci

Structure	Anatomy	Function
Intra-Articular		
ACL	Consists of 2 bundles that are parallel in extension and crossed in flexion[13,63]	Primary restraint against anterior tibial translation at all flexion angles, most pronounced at 30°[11] Secondary restraint against valgus[3]
Posterolateral bundle	Origin: medial aspect of lateral femoral condyle, distal to the bifurcate ridge Insertion: anterior aspect of the tibial plateau, posterior and lateral within the footprint	Taut in extension (higher in situ forces), tight during internal and external rotation[13,99]
Anteromedial bundle	Origin: medial aspect of lateral femoral condyle, proximal to the bifurcate ridge Insertion: anterior aspect of the tibial plateau, anterior and medial within the footprint	Taut in flexion (higher in situ forces)[99]
PCL	Origin: lateral aspect of the medial femoral condyle Insertion: posterior and inferior to the posterior rim of the tibial plateau	Primary restraint against posterior tibial translation at all flexion angles, most pronounced at flexion angles >20°[11,100,101] Secondary stabilizer against external rotation at high flexion angles only[3] No significant contribution to coronal stability
Posteromedial bundle	Origin: posterior and distal within the femoral origin Insertion: posterior and medial within the tibial footprint	Taut in extension[102,103]
Anterolateral bundle	Origin: anterior and proximal within the femoral origin Insertion: anterior and lateral within the tibial footprint	Taut in flexion[103] Higher stiffness and ultimate load than the PM bundle, but comparable in situ forces[102]
Meniscus	Medial meniscus: anteriorly attaches in front of the intermeniscal ligament, posteriorly attaches behind the medial tibial eminence, anterior to the PCL and medial to the articular cartilage margin[104,105] Lateral meniscus: anteriorly attaches immediately posterolateral to the ACL insertion; posteriorly it attaches just posterior to the lateral tibial eminence[104,105]	Important stabilizer against anteroposterior tibial translation in the cruciate-deficient knee[106]

The ACL and PCL have distinct bundles with synergistic functions.

Table 3
Extra-articular components of stability include the collateral ligaments, capsuloligamentous structures, popliteus, and iliotibial band

Structure	Anatomy	Function
Extra-articular		
Medial (tibial) collateral ligament		
Superficial	Origin: proximal and posterior to the medial epicondyle; anterior and distal to the adductor tubercle[107] Insertion: 6–8 mm from the joint line with a broad insertion of 2 separate pads that makes up the floor of the pes anserine bursa just anterior to the posteromedial crest of the tibia[107]	Primary stabilizer against valgus, most pronounced at 30° flexion[3] Primary stabilizer against internal rotation in flexion Secondary stabilizer against posterior translation in a PCL-deficient knee[3,16]
Deep	Origin: distal to the sMCL origin Insertion: just distal to the joint line, with attachments to the medial meniscus; can be described as meniscofemoral and meniscotibial portions[107]	Secondary stabilizer against valgus
Posterior oblique ligament	Origin: distal and posterior to the adductor tubercle Insertion: 3 separate arms insert on the posteromedial tibia, posteromedial capsule, and semimembranosus tendon[107]	Primary stabilizer against internal rotation in extension Secondary stabilizer against valgus and posterior drawer in full extension
Posteromedial capsule	Origin: posterior to the sMCL, tracking over the medial femoral condyle Insertion: posteromedial tibial rim	Secondary stabilizer against internal rotation[3]
Lateral (fibular) collateral ligament	Origin: slightly posterior and proximal to the lateral epicondyle Insertion: lateral aspect of the fibular head[9]	Primary stabilizer to varus from 0° to 30°, with less tension at higher flexion angles[10]
Posterolateral corner	Consists of the popliteus tendon, popliteofibular ligament, and fibular collateral ligament	Primary stabilizer against external rotation, most pronounced at 30° of flexion[3,8] Secondary stabilizer against varus load Secondary stabilizer to posterior tibial translation at low flexion angles[101]
Popliteus	Origin: posterior proximal tibia Insertion: posterior to the lateral femoral condyle articular margin, anterior, and distal to the LCL femoral origin[9]	Actively internally rotates the tibia Static stabilizer against external rotation and varus[9]

(continued on next page)

Table 3
(continued)

Structure	Anatomy	Function
Popliteofibular ligament	Origin: popliteus tendon Insertion: just anterior to the fibular styloid	Primary stabilizer against external rotation[3,7,94,108] Secondary stabilizer against varus and posterior translation
Iliotibial band	Origin: tensor fascia lata muscle Insertion: 2 femoral insertion sites (Kaplan fibers), one tibial insertion site (Gerdy's tubercle)[6]	Secondary stabilizer against tibial internal rotation in the ACL-deficient knee[6]
Anterolateral ligament	Origin: on the lateral epicondyle or posterosuperior to it Insertion: one band inserts onto the lateral meniscus, another inserts proximal to the biceps femoris tendon and has a variable relationship to the fibular collateral ligament insertion[5]	Secondary stabilizer to anterior tibial translation and internal rotation[4,5] Under most tension during 30° tibial internal rotation

Table 4
Articular components of stability include the tibial slope, coronal alignment of the knee, lateral femoral condyle ratio, and medial femoral condyle sphericity

Structure	Anatomy	Function
Articular		
Tibial slope	Physiologic normal tibial slope is approximately 11° (4°–13°)[109,110]	Increased posterior tibial slope may predispose to failure of ACL reconstruction by increasing anterior drawer forces[111,112] Decreased posterior tibial slope may have the same effect for PCL reconstructions by increasing posterior drawer forces[113,114]
Coronal alignment	Physiologic coronal alignment is approximately 9° of distal femoral valgus and 3° of proximal tibial varus[110] The resulting alignment is approximately 6° of cumulative valgus at the tibiofemoral joint	Varus alignment predisposes to failure of lateral reconstructions and ACL reconstructions[115] Valgus producing osteotomies can be used to treat posterolateral ligament injuries[116,117] Valgus alignment does not increase risk for revision ACL reconstruction[118]
Lateral femoral condyle ratio	Defines the anteroposterior depth of the lateral femoral condyle	Early retrospective data suggest a ratio >63% is associated with risk of ACL tear or failure of reconstruction[119]
Medial femoral condyle sphericity	Defined in a 3D MRI model by Lansdown and Ma.[120]	Increased sphericity is associated with persistently increased anterior tibial translations after ACL reconstruction[120,121]

- Simple translation occurs in the sagittal plane and causes pure anterior and posterior dislocation with cruciate ligament injury.
- Combining simple gaping and translation causes initial frontal gaping, followed by tibial translation to the opposite detached compartment. This results in peripheral ligament tearing at the convexity and detachment in the concavity with cruciate ligament disruption.
- Lastly, complex combined gaping and translation mechanisms cause double peripheral gaping, resulting in frontal and sagittal plane injuries in conjunction with rotation.

Mechanisms of Injury

- According Green and Allen,[23] the most common direction of dislocation is anterior (30%), then posterior (22%), lateral (15%), medial (4%), and rotatory (4.5%). The most common pattern of injury is a bicruciate ligament injury and, depending on the force direction, tears of the MCL or PLC.[24]
- The most common mechanism of an anterior dislocation is hyperextension of the knee.[23,25] Kennedy found the posterior capsule failed at 30° of hyperextension. At 50°, the ACL, PCL, and popliteal artery tore (with the caveat that vascular injury would occur with even less hyperextension in a live subject).[26]
- Hyperextension also results in the highest incidence of vascular injury because of the tethered nature of the popliteal artery and vein.[23]
- Posterior dislocations are usually high energy, as in a "dashboard" injury.[25]
- A varus injury mechanism causes a lateral dislocation and has the highest rate of associated peroneal nerve injury, due to the nerve being tethered near the fibular neck.[27]
- Valgus injury mechanism causes medial dislocations, however, most medial knee ligament tears are isolated and not multiligamentous injuries. These injuries occur predominantly in young individuals participating in sports activities, with the mechanism of injury involving valgus knee loading with external rotation.[28]
- A posterolateral knee dislocation results from a complex type mechanism causing ACL, PCL, and MCL tears with invagination into the knee joint. Buttonholing of the medial femoral condyle through the anteromedial capsule results in medial skin furrowing and risk of skin necrosis.[21,29] This can result in an inability to perform a closed reduction (**Fig. 1**).

Classification Systems

A knee dislocation can be simply described based on level of energy of the trauma, whether it is an open or closed injury, whether there was neurovascular injury, or if it is dislocated or subluxated. The higher energy mechanisms, such as motor vehicle accidents, have a higher incidence of vascular injuries.[30]

- The 2 main descriptive classification systems used for multiligamentous knee injuries and knee dislocations are Kennedy's and Schenck's.
- Kennedy's classification describes knee dislocation and is broken down into 5 types (anterior, posterior, lateral, medial, and rotatory) based on tibial displacement with respect to the rest of the knee.[26] The rotatory subtypes are anteromedial, anterolateral, posteromedial, and posterolateral.
  - Of the 22 dislocations from the original article, 14 were anterior, 2 posterior, 3 medial, and 3 lateral, with nerve or vascular involvement in over 50%.
  - Kennedy's classification is referred to as a position classification and was widely used. The main flaw with this system is that 50% of knee dislocations

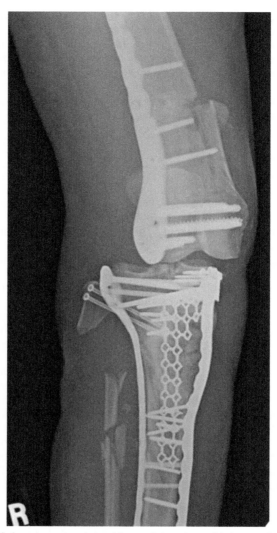

Fig. 1. Example of chronic posterolateral knee dislocation with button holing.

spontaneously reduced, and were unclassifiable using a positional classification system.[31]

- Schenck's anatomic classification of knee dislocations (KD) is based on the number of ligaments disrupted.[32,33] There are 5 major types, ranging from least ligamentous injury and lowest energy mechanism, to all ligaments with the highest energy mechanism.
  - KD I is classified as a knee dislocation with variable collateral involvement and either the PCL or ACL intact.
  - KD II is a bicruciate injury with intact collateral ligaments. Although rare, KD II injuries occur from a straight, hyperextended knee.[21]
  - KD III, with a subset of medial or lateral, has both cruciates torn with one collateral ligament torn.

- KD IV involves all of the cruciate and collateral ligaments tearing.
- KD V is a knee fracture dislocation.
- All contain subtypes C for arterial injury and N for neurologic injury.
- As described at the beginning of this section, the French Society of Orthopedic Surgery and Traumatology Symposium also created a pathophysiological classification, describing the direction of injury and pattern of ligament injury.[22]

BIOMECHANICS OF MLKI TREATMENT
Repair Versus Reconstruction

Considerable effort has been made to delineate which patients are most suited for repair versus reconstruction. Biomechanical literature regarding direct repair versus reconstruction in MLKI is sparse, and many decisions for reconstructive techniques are extrapolated from single or dual ligamentous injuries. In the event of a knee dislocation with MLKI, it is important to recognize that total biomechanical disruption of the knee joint is greater than the sum of its individual ligamentous injuries. Injury of effective static ligamentous restraints and the ensuing excessive demands on the dynamic stabilizers of the knee, lead to laxity in the knee, further compounding cartilaginous and meniscal damage.

- Richter and colleagues[34] evaluated 89 patients treated with traumatic KD, and compared ligamentous repair, reconstruction, and non-operative treatment. Not surprisingly, patients treated with either repair or reconstruction had improved outcome scores (Lysholm and Tegner scores) when compared with their non-operative counterparts. They add, however, that reconstruction in the instance of ligamentous avulsion repair is a viable alternative provided it is performed within 2 weeks of injury.
- Owens and colleagues[35] performed a retrospective review of 25 patients who sustained KD, and concluded that outcomes were similar for direct repair in patients with MLKI.
- In a meta-analysis of 9 studies, Frosch and colleagues[36] found conservative treatment of KD resulted in poor outcomes. Interestingly, the authors found comparable outcomes were seen with both direct suture repair versus reconstruction, without a finding a significant difference between the 2 treatment methods. In addition, they noted that the severity of the KD (eg, KD IV vs KD III) was more predictive of final outcome than the actual method of surgical treatment, with a higher KD level classification being more predictive of worse outcome. However, subsequent reviews and commentaries endorsed caution when using the direct repair approach to multiligament knee injuries.[37,38]
- With regard to the PLC, Stannard and colleagues[39] performed a non-randomized prospective study looking at repair versus reconstruction. Of these cases, 77% were MLIK. At 24 months follow-up, the authors found that repair had a failure rate of 37%, whereas reconstruction had a failure rate of only 9%.
- In a retrospective study, Levy and colleagues[40] corroborated these results by demonstrating a 40% failure rate with repairs and a 6% failure rate for reconstructions. LaPrade and colleagues[41] have also shown satisfactory results from their reconstruction technique, which functionally restores the fibular collateral ligament, popliteus tendon, and popliteofibular ligament.
- No biomechanical data studies have directly compared reconstruction and repair in the context of MLIK.

ACL

- There is a large body of literature demonstrating that ACL reconstruction is the gold standard technique for restoring anterior stability. From a biomechanical perspective, ACL reconstruction has proven itself with a variety of allograft and autograft options.[42,43]
- However, there is growing evidence that repair with augmentation may provide acceptable outcomes in some active patients.[44] In contrast, direct repair independent of augmentation has been shown to be inferior in an animal model and has a history of poor outcomes human models.[45,46]
- The ACL is commonly injured in the MLKI, usually in combination with the PCL and MCL.
- Tensioning of the PCL reconstruction may lead to increased tension seen at the ACL reconstruction, especially at high angle (>80°) tibial tunnels.[47]

PCL

- PCL reconstructions are often included in MLKI. Whereas isolated PCL injuries may otherwise be treated non-operatively with acceptable results, PCL-deficient knees show increased forces in both the medial and patellofemoral compartments.[48,49]
- With the secondary stabilizer injuries of the posterior knee (posterior joint capsule, PLC, hamstrings) that can occur with MLKI, reconstruction is indicated in the context of gross biomechanical disruption of the knee.[20,50]
- Consideration *must* be given to associated PLC injuries as well, with an intra-/pre-operative "dial" testing, and meticulous review of pre-operative advanced imaging.[51–53]
- Harner and colleagues[54] showed a 22% to 50% increase in forces across the PCL when the PLC was not reconstructed. LaPrade and colleagues[55] added to these findings: they found that coupled loading of posterior drawer force and external tibial torque at 30°, 60°, and 90° significantly increased force on the PCL graft. They also observed that failure to account for PLC injuries after reconstruction of the PCL leads to increased forces placed on the graft material. More recent literature has corroborated this evidence.[56,57]

Single Versus Double-Bundle ACL and PCL

- Given the biomechanical complexity of MLI, the treating surgeon should be prepared to use a variety of repair, reconstructive, and staged techniques. An important caveat is that all strands of a soft tissue graft—particularly hamstrings—must be under similar tension to maximize tensile properties of the graft.[58,59]
- An important consideration in MLKI is tunnel placement. Whereas anatomic reconstruction may confer a biomechanical advantage, available bone in the proximal tibia and distal femur may be a limiting factor.[60–62]
- Yagi and colleagues[63] produced a pivotal biomechanical article that evaluated anterior forces versus combined anterior and rotary forces on ACL-deficient, single-bundle (SB), and anatomic (DB) ACL reconstruction. They found that the anatomic/double-bundle repair more closely resembled the intact cruciate ligament model against both anterior and rotatory forces; finding it to normalize in situ forces to the intact model 97% ± 9% and 91% ± 35%, respectively. While these findings have been corroborated, clinical results have not shown a difference.
- Double-bundle PCL reconstructions have gained momentum as a biomechanically superior technique as well, although this remains controversial.[59,64] While

studies by Markolf and colleagues[65] and Bergfeld and colleagues[66] showed no difference between SB and DB reconstructions, more recent data have argued otherwise. Double-bundle constructs tested in cadaveric specimens have shown to be biomechanically superior in deep flexion,[67] and that the anterolateral and posteromedial bundles play a codominant role necessitating individual reconstruction.[68]

- Two obstacles exist when applying the double-bundle techniques to MLKI. First, bone stock in both the distal femur and proximal tibia may be limited with multiple grafts, and convergent tunnels may ultimately weaken any one construct.[61,62] Secondly, much of the biomechanical data to SB or DB does not incorporate the additional dynamic knee stabilizer damage that occurs at time of injury in an MLKI. Surgeons should be prepared to sacrifice a potentially biomechanically superior approach if multiple grafts provide more reproducible knee kinematics.

MCL

- MCL damage is common in KD.[69]
- MCL avulsions are commonly off of the femoral origin.
- The surgeon may address medial knee injury with a variety of options:
  - Bracing—usually reserved for partial tears (grade I or II) with *anatomic* restoration of the remaining ligamentous and capsular relationships,[70]
  - Direct repair both with and without augmentation, and
  - Hamstring allograft reconstruction, which may be as a single or double bundle.[71,72]
- Augmented repair of the MCL with internal bracing has promising, albeit contested results. Wijdicks and colleagues[73] found no difference between augmented and non-augmented sMCL repairs at time zero under valgus and rotary testing in fresh frozen cadavers. Both were biomechanically inferior to the intact state. More recent data from Gilmer and colleagues (described below) may yield promising results moving forward.
- PMC injuries, which often coincide with MCL injuries in MLKI, must be addressed as well. Numerous reconstructive techniques have been described.[70,72]
- Ultimately, the surgeon should maintain a high suspicion for MCL injury in MLKI. Whereas no one reconstructive method has shown superiority in the context of a knee dislocation or MLKI, careful consideration must be given to increased loads at the ACL, PMC, and menisci with valgus laxity.
- Similar to PCL injuries, MCL reconstruction or repair is indicated acutely following MLKI.[28,74,75]
- In a systematic review of 8 studies looking at medial-sided repair versus reconstruction, Kovachevich and colleagues[75] found satisfactory outcomes with both procedures. Unfortunately, none of the included studies were prospective. They also found no prospective studies of surgical versus non-surgical management of these medial injuries.

LCL

- LCL surgical treatments include repair, reconstruction, and tenodesis of the biceps femoris tendon.[76]
  - Isolated LCL reconstructions can restore varus and rotational stability in the absence of other lateral sided injuries.[77]
  - However, when addressing the lateral side of the knee, it is important to reconstruct all injured structures. McCarthy and colleagues[78] compared reconstruction of the LCL and popliteus with reconstruction of the LCL, popliteus, and

popliteofibular ligament. They found that failure to reconstruct the PFL resulted in increased varus translation at lower flexion angles, and increased internal rotation laxity at higher flexion angles.

○ Similarly, Markolf and colleagues[79] found that reconstruction of the LCL alone did not adequately restore external rotation stability. This placed added stress on PCL reconstructions in their cadaver model. The addition of PFL and popliteus reconstructions restored PCL graft forces to within normal limits.

○ Care must be taken not to cause varus over-constraint, which is possible with these reconstructions.[80]

INTERNAL BRACING

• Recently, the concept of adding an "internal brace" with the use of an ultra-high molecular-weight polyethylene/polyester tape to bridge the graft has grown in popularity.[81] The goal of these devices is to provide a stable, load-sharing implant during the critical first 6 months of healing.[82] Ideally, augmentations of graft material or ligamentous repairs with internal bracing should allow patients to return to weight bearing sooner with rapid return to range of motion postoperatively. A recent review by van Eck and colleagues[81] revealed that the literature supports favorable post-operative outcomes as well.

• While further biomechanical data on "internal bracing," or "suture augmentation," for the PCL are pending, promising biomechanical results exist for repair and reconstruction of the ACL and MCL.

○ Gilmer and colleagues[83] reviewed MCL reconstruction, repair with internal bracing, and intact cadaver MCLs with moment to failure as the primary endpoint. They found MCL repair with internal bracing to be similar to reconstruction for moment to failure, and whereas both were superior to repair alone, they were both inferior to the intact state.

○ Bachmaier and colleagues[84] studied ACL internal bracing in a full construct model. They found that reinforcement of small diameter hamstring tendon grafts reduced elongation of the graft by 38%, with a 64% increase in ultimate failure load. They concluded that this technique can improve graft stability without stress-shielding the tissue.

○ Fisher and colleagues[85] evaluated restoration of native joint biomechanics with the use of suture augmentation in the goat stifle joint, which mimics the human knee joint. Using 2 sutures and suspensory fixation construct, they found that anterior tibial translation was within 3 mm to the intact state when internal bracing was added to the ACL repair. The investigators also found a reduced load on the medial meniscus—an important secondary sagittal stabilizer—when using this construct.

SUMMARY

• The knee has 6° of freedom that necessitate stability in the coronal, sagittal, and axial planes.

• Primary stabilizers in the coronal plane are the superficial MCL and the lateral (fibular) collateral ligament.

• Primary stabilizers in the sagittal plane are the anterior and PCLs.

• Primary stabilizers in the rotational plane are the POL, superficial MCL, LCL, and PLC structures.

• Secondary stabilizers are increasingly important in the case of injury to multiple primary stabilizers.

- Repair or reconstruction of all significantly injured structures has the best chance of restoring biomechanics and preventing persistent laxity.
- Classification systems for MLKI can be useful in describing the pathomechanics or severity of injury.
- Whereas biomechanics research of individual ligament injuries is abundant, there is a paucity of direct biomechanical data on multiple ligament injuries. Applying existing data to MLI patients can be helpful, but more direct research is needed.

REFERENCES

1. Woo SL-Y, Debski RE, Withrow JD, et al. Biomechanics of knee ligaments. Am J Sports Med 1999;27(4):533–43.
2. Grood ES, Suntay WJ. A joint coordinate system for the clinical description of three-dimensional motions: application to the knee. J Biomech Eng 1983; 105(2):136.
3. Amis AA, Bull AMJ, Gupte CM, et al. Biomechanics of the PCL and related structures: posterolateral, posteromedial and meniscofemoral ligaments. Knee Surg Sports Traumatol Arthrosc 2003;11(5):271–81.
4. Kennedy MI, Claes S, Fuso FAF, et al. The anterolateral ligament. Am J Sports Med 2015;43(7):1606–15.
5. Kraeutler MJ, Welton KL, Chahla J, et al. Current concepts of the anterolateral ligament of the knee: anatomy, biomechanics, and reconstruction. Am J Sports Med 2017. https://doi.org/10.1177/0363546517701920. 36354651770192.
6. Godin JA, Chahla J, Moatshe G, et al. A comprehensive reanalysis of the distal iliotibial band: quantitative anatomy, radiographic markers, and biomechanical properties. Am J Sports Med 2017;45(11):2595–603.
7. Terry GC, LaPrade RF. The posterolateral aspect of the knee. Am J Sports Med 1996;24(6):732–9.
8. Gollehon DL, Torzilli PA, Warren RF. The role of the posterolateral and cruciate ligaments in the stability of the human knee. A biomechanical study. J Bone Joint Surg Am 1987;69(2):233–42.
9. Sanchez AR, Sugalski MT, LaPrade RF. Anatomy and biomechanics of the lateral side of the knee. Sports Med Arthrosc Rev 2006;14(1):2–11.
10. LaPrade RF, Wentorf F. Diagnosis and treatment of posterolateral knee injuries. Clin Orthop Relat Res 2002;(402):110–21.
11. Butler DL, Noyes FR, Grood ES. Ligamentous restraints to anterior-posterior drawer in the human knee. A biomechanical study. J Bone Joint Surg Am 1980;62(2):259–70.
12. Pensy RA, Brunton LM, Parks BG, et al. Single-incision extensile volar approach to the distal radius and concurrent carpal tunnel release: cadaveric study. J Hand Surg Am 2010;35(2):217–22.
13. Chhabra A. Anatomic, radiographic, biomechanical, and kinematic evaluation of the anterior cruciate ligament and its two functional bundles. J Bone Joint Surg Am 2006;88(suppl_4):2.
14. Li G, Gill TJ, DeFrate LE, et al. Biomechanical consequences of PCL deficiency in the knee under simulated muscle loads - an in vitro experimental study. J Orthop Res 2002;20(4):887–92.
15. Voos JE, Mauro CS, Wente T, et al. Posterior cruciate ligament. Am J Sports Med 2012;40(1):222–31.

16. Ritchie JR, Bergfeld JA, Kambic H, et al. Isolated sectioning of the medial and posteromedial capsular ligaments in the posterior cruciate ligament-deficient knee. Am J Sports Med 1998;26(3):389–94.

17. LaPrade RF, Resig S, Wentorf F, et al. The effects of grade III posterolateral knee complex injuries on anterior cruciate ligament graft force. Am J Sports Med 1999;27(4):469–75.

18. Battaglia MJ, Lenhoff MW, Ehteshami JR, et al. Medial collateral ligament injuries and subsequent load on the anterior cruciate ligament: a biomechanical evaluation in a cadaveric model. Am J Sports Med 2009;37(2):305–11.

19. Woodmass JM, O'Malley MP, Krych AJ, et al. Revision multiligament knee reconstruction: clinical outcomes and proposed treatment algorithm. Arthroscopy 2017;1–9. https://doi.org/10.1016/j.arthro.2017.09.022.

20. Levy BA, Dajani KA, Whelan DB, et al. Decision making in the multiligament-injured knee: an evidence-based systematic review. Arthroscopy 2009;25(4): 430–8.

21. Schenck RC, Richter DL, Wascher DC. Knee dislocations: lessons learned from 20-year follow-up. Orthop J Sports Med 2014;2(5). 2325967114534387.

22. Boisgard S, Versier G, Descamps S, et al. Bicruciate ligament lesions and dislocation of the knee: mechanisms and classification. Orthop Traumatol Surg Res 2009;95(8):627–31.

23. Green NE, Allen BL. Vascular injuries associated with dislocation of the knee. J Bone Joint Surg Am 1977;59(2):236–9. Available at: http://www.ncbi.nlm.nih.gov/pubmed/845209.

24. Robertson A, Nutton RW, Keating JF. Dislocation of the knee. J Bone Joint Surg Br 2006;88(6):706–11.

25. Rihn JA, Groff YJ, Harner CD, et al. The acutely dislocated knee: evaluation and management. J Am Acad Orthop Surg 2004;12(5):334–46. Available at: http://www.ncbi.nlm.nih.gov/pubmed/15469228.

26. Kennedy JC. Complete dislocation of the knee joint. J Bone Joint Surg Am 1963; 45:889–904. Available at: http://www.ncbi.nlm.nih.gov/pubmed/14046474.

27. Niall DM. Palsy of the common peroneal nerve after traumatic dislocation of the knee. J Bone Joint Surg Br 2005;87-B(5):664–7.

28. Wijdicks CA, Griffith CJ, Johansen S, et al. Injuries to the medial collateral ligament and associated medial structures of the knee. J Bone Joint Surg Am 2010; 92(5):1266–80.

29. Quinlan AG, Sharrard WJ. Postero-lateral dislocation of the knee with capsular interposition. J Bone Joint Surg Br 1958;40-B(4):660–3. Available at: http://www.ncbi.nlm.nih.gov/pubmed/13610979.

30. Fanelli GC, Orcutt DR, Edson CJ. The multiple-ligament injured knee: evaluation, treatment, and results. Arthroscopy 2005;21(4):471–86.

31. Wascher DC, Dvirnak PC, DeCoster TA. Knee dislocation: initial assessment and implications for treatment. J Orthop Trauma 1997;11(7):525–9. Available at: http://www.ncbi.nlm.nih.gov/pubmed/9334955.

32. Schenck RC. The dislocated knee. Instr Course Lect 1994;43:127–36. Available at: http://www.ncbi.nlm.nih.gov/pubmed/9097143.

33. Walker D, Hardison R, Schenck RJ. A baker's dozen of knee dislocations. Am J Knee Surg 1994;7:117–24.

34. Richter M, Bosch U, Wippermann B, et al. Comparison of surgical repair or reconstruction of the cruciate ligaments versus nonsurgical treatment in patients with traumatic knee dislocations. Am J Sports Med 2002;30(5):718–27.

35. Owens BD, Neault M, Benson E, et al. Primary repair of knee dislocations: results in 25 patients (28 knees) at a mean follow-up of four years. J Orthop Trauma 2007;21(2):92–6.
36. Frosch K-H, Preiss A, Heider S, et al. Primary ligament sutures as a treatment option of knee dislocations: a meta-analysis. Knee Surg Sports Traumatol Arthrosc 2013;21(7):1502–9.
37. Levy BA, Fanelli GC, Whelan DB, et al. Controversies in the treatment of knee dislocations and multiligament reconstruction. J Am Acad Orthop Surg 2009; 17(4):197–206. Available at: http://www.ncbi.nlm.nih.gov/pubmed/19307669.
38. Miller MD. Re: primary repair of knee dislocations: results in 25 patients (28 knees) at a mean follow-up of four years. J Orthop Trauma 2007;21(2):97 [discussion: 97–8].
39. Stannard JP, Brown SL, Farris RC, et al. The posterolateral corner of the knee: repair versus reconstruction. Am J Sports Med 2005;33(6):881–8.
40. Levy BA, Dajani KA, Morgan JA, et al. Repair versus reconstruction of the fibular collateral ligament and posterolateral corner in the multiligament-injured knee. Am J Sports Med 2010;38(4):804–9.
41. LaPrade RF, Johansen S, Agel J, et al. Outcomes of an anatomic posterolateral knee reconstruction. J Bone Joint Surg Am 2010;92(1):16–22.
42. Mascarenhas R, MacDonald PB. Anterior cruciate ligament reconstruction: a look at prosthetics–past, present and possible future. Mcgill J Med 2008;11(1):29–37. Available at: http://www.ncbi.nlm.nih.gov/pmc/articles/PMC2322926/ http://www.ncbi.nlm.nih.gov/pmc/articles/PMC2322926/pdf/mjm11_1p29.pdf.
43. Seitz H, Menth-Chiari WA, Lang S, et al. Histological evaluation of the healing potential of the anterior cruciate ligament by means of augmented and non-augmented repair: an in vivo animal study. Knee Surg Sports Traumatol Arthrosc 2008;16(12):1087–93.
44. van der List JP, DiFelice GS. Preservation of the anterior cruciate ligament: surgical techniques. Am J Orthop (Belle Mead NJ) 2016;45(7):E406–14. Available at: http://www.ncbi.nlm.nih.gov/pubmed/28005094.
45. Feagin JA, Curl WW. Isolated tear of the anterior cruciate ligament: 5-year followup study. Clin Orthop Relat Res 1996;325:4–9. Available at: http://www.ncbi.nlm.nih.gov/pubmed/8998897.
46. Taylor DC, Posner M, Curl WW, et al. Isolated tears of the anterior cruciate ligament: over 30-year follow-up of patients treated with arthrotomy and primary repair. Am J Sports Med 2009;37(1):65–71.
47. Simmons R, Howell SM, Hull ML. Effect of the angle of the femoral and tibial tunnels in the coronal plane and incremental excision of the posterior cruciate ligament on tension of an anterior cruciate ligament graft: an in vitro study. J Bone Joint Surg Am 2003;85-A(6):1018–29. http://www.ncbi.nlm.nih.gov/pubmed/12783997.
48. Logan M, Williams A, Lavelle J, et al. The effect of posterior cruciate ligament deficiency on knee kinematics. Am J Sports Med 2004;32(8):1915–22. Available at: http://www.ncbi.nlm.nih.gov/pubmed/15572321.
49. MacDonald P, Miniaci A, Fowler P, et al. A biomechanical analysis of joint contact forces in the posterior cruciate deficient knee. Knee Surg Sports Traumatol Arthrosc 1996;3(4):252–5. Available at: http://www.ncbi.nlm.nih.gov/pubmed/8739723.
50. Wind WM, Bergfeld JA, Parker RD. Evaluation and treatment of posterior cruciate ligament injuries. Am J Sports Med 2004;32(7):1765–75.

51. Bae JH, Choi IC, Suh SW, et al. Evaluation of the reliability of the dial test for posterolateral rotatory instability: a cadaveric study using an isotonic rotation machine. Arthroscopy 2008;24(5):593–8.

52. Ranawat A, Baker CL, Henry S, et al. Posterolateral corner injury of the knee: evaluation and management. J Am Acad Orthop Surg 2008;16(9):506–18. Available at: http://www.ncbi.nlm.nih.gov/pubmed/18768708.

53. Twaddle BC, Hunter JC, Chapman JR, et al. MRI in acute knee dislocation. A prospective study of clinical, MRI, and surgical findings. J Bone Joint Surg Br 1996;78(4):573–9. Available at: http://www.ncbi.nlm.nih.gov/pubmed/8682823.

54. Harner CD, Vogrin TM, Höher J, et al. Biomechanical analysis of a posterior cruciate ligament reconstruction. Deficiency of the posterolateral structures as a cause of graft failure. Am J Sports Med 2000;28(1):32–9.

55. LaPrade RF, Muench C, Wentorf F, et al. The effect of injury to the posterolateral structures of the knee on force in a posterior cruciate ligament graft. Am J Sports Med 2002;30(2):233–8.

56. Chahla J, Moatshe G, Dean CS, et al. Posterolateral corner of the knee: current concepts. Arch Bone Jt Surg 2016;4(2):97–103. Available at: http://www.ncbi.nlm.nih.gov/pubmed/27200384.

57. Lunden JB, Bzdusek PJ, Monson JK, et al. Current concepts in the recognition and treatment of posterolateral corner injuries of the knee. J Orthop Sports Phys Ther 2010;40(8):502–16.

58. Hamner DL, Brown CH, Steiner ME, et al. Hamstring tendon grafts for reconstruction of the anterior cruciate ligament: biomechanical evaluation of the use of multiple strands and tensioning techniques. J Bone Joint Surg Am 1999; 81(4):549–57. Available at: http://www.ncbi.nlm.nih.gov/pubmed/10225801.

59. Markolf KL, Feeley BT, Jackson SR, et al. Biomechanical studies of double-bundle posterior cruciate ligament reconstructions. J Bone Jt Surg 2006; 88(8):1788–94.

60. Hussein M, van Eck CF, Cretnik A, et al. Prospective randomized clinical evaluation of conventional single-bundle, anatomic single-bundle, and anatomic double-bundle anterior cruciate ligament reconstruction: 281 cases with 3- to 5-year follow-up. Am J Sports Med 2012;40(3):512–20.

61. Moatshe G, Slette EL, Engebretsen L, et al. Intertunnel relationships in the tibia during reconstruction of multiple knee ligaments: how to avoid tunnel convergence. Am J Sports Med 2016;44(11):2864–9.

62. Moatshe G, Brady AW, Slette EL, et al. Multiple ligament reconstruction femoral tunnels: intertunnel relationships and guidelines to avoid convergence. Am J Sports Med 2017;45(3):563–9.

63. Yagi M, Wong EK, Kanamori A, et al. Biomechanical analysis of an anatomic anterior cruciate ligament reconstruction. Am J Sports Med 2002;30(5):660–6.

64. Tucker CJ, Joyner PW, Endres NK. Single versus double-bundle PCL reconstruction: scientific rationale and clinical evidence. Curr Rev Musculoskelet Med 2018;11(2):285–9.

65. Markolf KL, Jackson SR, McAllister DR. Single- versus double-bundle posterior cruciate ligament reconstruction: effects of femoral tunnel separation. Am J Sports Med 2010;38(6):1141–6.

66. Bergfeld JA, Graham SM, Parker RD, et al. A biomechanical comparison of posterior cruciate ligament reconstructions using single- and double-bundle tibial inlay techniques. Am J Sports Med 2005;33(7):976–81.

67. Wijdicks CA, Kennedy NI, Goldsmith MT, et al. Kinematic analysis of the posterior cruciate ligament, part 2: a comparison of anatomic single- versus double-bundle reconstruction. Am J Sports Med 2013;41(12):2839–48.

68. Kennedy NI, Wijdicks CA, Goldsmith MT, et al. Kinematic analysis of the posterior cruciate ligament, part 1: the individual and collective function of the anterolateral and posteromedial bundles. Am J Sports Med 2013;41(12):2828–38.

69. Harner CD, Waltrip RL, Bennett CH, et al. Surgical management of knee dislocations. J Bone Joint Surg Am 2004;86-A(2):262–73. Available at: http://www.ncbi.nlm.nih.gov/pubmed/14960670.

70. Lachman JR, Rehman S, Pipitone PS. Traumatic knee dislocations: evaluation, management, and surgical treatment. Orthop Clin North Am 2015;46(4):479–93.

71. Kitamura N, Ogawa M, Kondo E, et al. A novel medial collateral ligament reconstruction procedure using semitendinosus tendon autograft in patients with multiligamentous knee injuries. Am J Sports Med 2013;41(6):1274–81.

72. Borden PS, Kantaras AT, Caborn DNM. Medial collateral ligament reconstruction with allograft using a double-bundle technique. Arthroscopy 2002;18(4):E19. Available at: http://www.ncbi.nlm.nih.gov/pubmed/11951187.

73. Wijdicks CA, Michalski MP, Rasmussen MT, et al. Superficial medial collateral ligament anatomic augmented repair versus anatomic reconstruction: an in vitro biomechanical analysis. Am J Sports Med 2013;41(12):2858–66.

74. Tibor LM, Marchant MH, Taylor DC, et al. Management of medial-sided knee injuries, part 2: posteromedial corner. Am J Sports Med 2011;39(6):1332–40.

75. Kovachevich R, Shah JP, Arens AM, et al. Operative management of the medial collateral ligament in the multi-ligament injured knee: an evidence-based systematic review. Knee Surg Sports Traumatol Arthrosc 2009;17(7):823–9.

76. Grawe B, Schroeder AJ, Kakazu R, et al. Lateral collateral ligament injury about the knee: anatomy, evaluation, and management. J Am Acad Orthop Surg 2018;26(6):e120–7.

77. Liu P, Wang J, Zhao F, et al. Anatomic, arthroscopically assisted, mini-open fibular collateral ligament reconstruction: an in vitro biomechanical study. Am J Sports Med 2014;42(2):373–81.

78. McCarthy M, Camarda L, Wijdicks CA, et al. Anatomic posterolateral knee reconstructions require a popliteofibular ligament reconstruction through a tibial tunnel. Am J Sports Med 2010;38(8):1674–81.

79. Markolf KL, Graves BR, Sigward SM, et al. Effects of posterolateral reconstructions on external tibial rotation and forces in a posterior cruciate ligament graft. J Bone Joint Surg Am 2007;89(11):2351–8.

80. Markolf KL, Graves BR, Sigward SM, et al. How well do anatomical reconstructions of the posterolateral corner restore varus stability to the posterior cruciate ligament-reconstructed knee? Am J Sports Med 2007;35(7):1117–22.

81. van Eck CF, Limpisvasti O, ElAttrache NS. Is there a role for internal bracing and repair of the anterior cruciate ligament? a systematic literature review. Am J Sports Med 2017. https://doi.org/10.1177/0363546517717956. 36354651771795.

82. Hanley P, Lew WD, Lewis JL, et al. Load sharing and graft forces in anterior cruciate ligament reconstructions with the ligament augmentation device. Am J Sports Med 1989;17(3):414–22.

83. Gilmer BB, Crall T, DeLong J, et al. Biomechanical analysis of internal bracing for treatment of medial knee injuries. Orthopedics 2016;39(3):e532–7.

84. Bachmaier S, Smith PA, Bley J, et al. Independent suture tape reinforcement of small and standard diameter grafts for anterior cruciate ligament reconstruction: a biomechanical full construct model. Arthroscopy 2018;34(2):490–9.

85. Fisher MB, Jung H-J, McMahon PJ, et al. Suture augmentation following ACL injury to restore the function of the ACL, MCL, and medial meniscus in the goat stifle joint. J Biomech 2011;44(8):1530–5.

86. Geeslin AG, Chahla J, Moatshe G, et al. Anterolateral knee extra-articular stabilizers: a robotic sectioning study of the anterolateral ligament and distal iliotibial band kaplan fibers. Am J Sports Med 2018;46(6):1352–61.

87. Noyes FR, Huser LE, Levy MS. Rotational knee instability in ACL-deficient knees: role of the anterolateral ligament and iliotibial band as defined by tibiofemoral compartment translations and rotations. J Bone Joint Surg Am 2017;99(4): 305–14.

88. Zaffagnini S, Signorelli C, Bonanzinga T, et al. Does meniscus removal affect ACL-deficient knee laxity? An in vivo study. Knee Surg Sports Traumatol Arthrosc 2016;24(11):3599–604.

89. Shoemaker SC, Markolf KL. The role of the meniscus in the anterior-posterior stability of the loaded anterior cruciate-deficient knee. Effects of partial versus total excision. J Bone Joint Surg Am 1986;68(1):71–9. Available at: http://www.ncbi.nlm.nih.gov/pubmed/3753605.

90. DePhillipo NN, Moatshe G, Brady A, et al. Effect of meniscocapsular and meniscotibial lesions in ACL-deficient and ACL-reconstructed knees: a biomechanical study. Am J Sports Med 2018. https://doi.org/10.1177/0363546518774315. 363546518774315.

91. Frank JM, Moatshe G, Brady AW, et al. Lateral meniscus posterior root and meniscofemoral ligaments as stabilizing structures in the ACL-deficient knee: a biomechanical study. Orthop J Sports Med 2017;5(6). https://doi.org/10.1177/2325967117695756.

92. Petersen W, Loerch S, Schanz S, et al. The role of the posterior oblique ligament in controlling posterior tibial translation in the posterior cruciate ligament-deficient knee. Am J Sports Med 2008;36(3):495–501.

93. Gupte CM, Bull AMJ, Thomas RD, et al. The meniscofemoral ligaments: secondary restraints to the posterior drawer. Analysis of anteroposterior and rotary laxity in the intact and posterior-cruciate-deficient knee. J Bone Joint Surg Br 2003; 85(5):765–73. Available at: http://www.ncbi.nlm.nih.gov/pubmed/12892207.

94. Veltri DM, Deng XH, Torzilli PA, et al. The role of the popliteofibular ligament in stability of the human knee. A biomechanical study. Am J Sports Med 1995; 24(1):19–27.

95. Nielsen S, Helmig P. The static stabilizing function of the popliteal tendon in the knee. An experimental study. Arch Orthop Trauma Surg 1986;104(6):357–62. Available at: http://www.ncbi.nlm.nih.gov/pubmed/3964042.

96. Warren LA, Marshall JL, Girgis F. The prime static stabilizer of the medial side of the knee. J Bone Joint Surg Am 1974;56(4):665–74. Available at: http://www.ncbi.nlm.nih.gov/pubmed/4835814.

97. LaPrade MD, Kennedy MI, Wijdicks CA, et al. Anatomy and biomechanics of the medial side of the knee and their surgical implications. Sports Med Arthrosc Rev 2015;23(2):63–70.

98. Haimes JL, Wroble RR, Grood ES, et al. Role of the medial structures in the intact and anterior cruciate ligament-deficient knee. Am J Sports Med 1994; 22(3):402–9.

99. Sakane M, Fox RJ, Woo SLY, et al. In situ forces in the anterior cruciate ligament and its bundles in response to anterior tibial loads. J Orthop Res 1997;15(2): 285–93.

100. Amis AA, Jakob RP. Anterior cruciate ligament graft positioning, tensioning and twisting. Knee Surg Sports Traumatol Arthrosc 1998;6(Suppl 1):S2–12.

101. Grood ES, Stowers SF, Noyes FR. Limits of movement in the human knee. Effect of sectioning the posterior cruciate ligament and posterolateral structures. J Bone Joint Surg Am 1988;70(1):88–97.

102. Fox RJ, Harner CD, Sakane M, et al. Determination of the in situ forces in the human posterior cruciate ligament using robotic technology: a cadaveric study. Am J Sports Med 1998;26(3):395–401.

103. Harner CD, Xerogeanes JW, Livesay GA, et al. The human posterior cruciate ligament complex: an interdisciplinary study. Am J Sports Med 1995;23(6):736–45.

104. LaPrade CM, Ellman MB, Rasmussen MT, et al. Anatomy of the anterior root attachments of the medial and lateral menisci. Am J Sports Med 2014;42(10): 2386–92.

105. Johannsen AM, Civitarese DM, Padalecki JR, et al. Qualitative and quantitative anatomic analysis of the posterior root attachments of the medial and lateral menisci. Am J Sports Med 2012;40(10):2342–7.

106. Allen CR, Wong EK, Livesay GA, et al. Importance of the medial meniscus in the anterior cruciate ligament-deficient knee. J Orthop Res 2000;18(1):109–15.

107. LaPrade RF. The anatomy of the medial part of the knee. J Bone Jt Surg 2007; 89(9):2000.

108. LaPrade RF, Terry GC. Injuries to the posterolateral aspect of the knee. Am J Sports Med 1997;25(4):433–8.

109. Ho JPY, Merican AM, Hashim MS, et al. Three-dimensional computed tomography analysis of the posterior tibial slope in 100 knees. J Arthroplasty 2017; 32(10):3176–83.

110. Luo CF. Reference axes for reconstruction of the knee. Knee 2004;11(4):251–7.

111. Shelburne KB, Kim HJ, Sterett WI, et al. Effect of posterior tibial slope on knee biomechanics during functional activity. J Orthop Res 2011;29(2):223–31.

112. Salmon LJ, Heath E, Akrawi H, et al. 20-year outcomes of anterior cruciate ligament reconstruction with hamstring tendon autograft: the catastrophic effect of age and posterior tibial slope. Am J Sports Med 2017. https://doi.org/10. 1177/0363546517741497. 36354651774149.

113. Gwinner C, Weiler A, Roider M, et al. Tibial slope strongly influences knee stability after posterior cruciate ligament reconstruction: a prospective 5- to 15-year follow-up. Am J Sports Med 2017;45(2):355–61.

114. Giffin JR, Stabile KJ, Zantop T, et al. Importance of tibial slope for stability of the posterior cruciate ligament deficient knee. Am J Sports Med 2007;35(9):1443–9.

115. Won HH, Chang CB, Je MS, et al. Coronal limb alignment and indications for high tibial osteotomy in patients undergoing revision ACL reconstruction. Clin Orthop Relat Res 2013;471(11):3504–11.

116. Arthur A, LaPrade RF, Agel J. Proximal tibial opening wedge osteotomy as the initial treatment for chronic posterolateral corner deficiency in the varus knee: a prospective clinical study. Am J Sports Med 2007;35(11):1844–50.

117. Tischer T, Paul J, Pape D, et al. The impact of osseous malalignment and realignment procedures in knee ligament surgery: a systematic review of the clinical evidence. Orthop J Sports Med 2017;5(3). 2325967117697287.

118. Mitchell JJ, Cinque ME, Dornan GJ, et al. Primary versus revision anterior cruciate ligament reconstruction: patient demographics, radiographic findings, and associated lesions. Arthroscopy 2018;34(3):695–703.
119. Pfeiffer TR, Burnham JM, Hughes JD, et al. An increased lateral femoral condyle ratio is a risk factor for anterior cruciate ligament injury. J Bone Jt Surg 2018; 100(10):857–64.
120. Lansdown D, Ma CB. The influence of tibial and femoral bone morphology on knee kinematics in the anterior cruciate ligament injured knee. Clin Sports Med 2018;37(1):127–36.
121. Lansdown DA, Pedoia V, Zaid M, et al. Variations in knee kinematics after ACL injury and after reconstruction are correlated with bone shape differences. Clin Orthop Relat Res 2017;475(10):2427–35.

Multiligament Knee Injury
Injury Patterns, Outcomes, and Gait Analysis

Thomas Neri, MD, PhD*, Darli Myat, PhD, Aaron Beach, PhD,
David Anthony Parker, BMedSci, MBBS, FRACS, FAOrthA

KEYWORDS

- Knee • Multiligament injury • Injury patterns • Outcomes • Gait analysis

KEY POINTS

- High-velocity traumatism, such as road accidents and sporting activities, has been reported as the main injury mechanism of multiligament knee injury (MLKI).
- A combination of 1 cruciate tear with a medial or lateral side injury is the most frequent injury pattern.
- Associated lesions, such as neurovascular and meniscal injuries, are frequently combined with MLKI and should be considered during injury assessment.
- Regardless of the injury severity, the functional and clinical outcomes demonstrate that MLKIs have a significant impact on knee function and patients rarely return to normal after treatment.
- Although gait differences are patient-specific, multiligament knee reconstruction patients displayed significant alterations in knee kinematics and spatiotemporal gait characteristics not identified in healthy controls during walking.

INTRODUCTION

Multiligament knee injuries (MLKIs) involve complete injury to a combination of at least 2 of the 4 major ligaments: anterior cruciate ligament (ACL), posterior cruciate ligament (PCL), medial collateral ligament (MCL), and/or posterolateral corner (PLC). Although rare, with an incidence of 0.002% to 0.2% per year, MLKIs are potentially devastating.[1,2] Although there are various mechanisms for injury, MLKIs are most commonly the consequence of a knee dislocation (KD) due to a high-energy trauma, such as motor vehicle accident or sports injury. This high-velocity injury can occur in polytrauma patients or in isolation.[3] Not as common, but well recognized, are ultra–low-velocity dislocations of the knee, which may be

---

Disclosure Statement: No Disclosure of any relationship with a commercial company for all authors.
Sydney Orthopaedic Research Institute (SORI), Level 1, The Gallery 445 Victoria Avenue, Chatswood, New South Wales 2067, Australia
* Corresponding author.
E-mail address: tneri@sori.com.au

https://doi.org/10.1016/j.csm.2018.11.010
0278-5919/19/© 2018 Elsevier Inc. All rights reserved.
sportsmed.theclinics.com

associated with overload in superobese patients.[4] Regardless of the cause, because MLKI dislocations often reduce spontaneously, the incidence may be underestimated.[5] Consequently, MLKIs are difficult to study. Management of these injuries is still challenging and many questions remain unresolved.[6] What is the distribution of the injury pattern and the incidence of associated complications? What clinical outcomes can a patient expect after surgery to address an MLKI? Does a multiligament knee reconstruction (MLKR) restore normal knee kinematics with a physiologic gait?

One of the major difficulties in dealing with MLKIs is the varying patterns of ligamentous disruption that fall under this broad heading. There are many possible combinations that could be classified as an MLKI.[1,7] This is without considering other factors, such as the complication of additional injuries to other structures of the knee. During a KD, peroneal nerve[8,9] and popliteal artery[10,11] injuries can happen. In addition, fracture,[12] chondral damage, meniscal tears,[13] and residual laxity in a dislocated knee can lead to early-onset osteoarthritis.[14] Nevertheless, the respective incidence of these associated lesions remains unknown because the literature is usually based on a registry database or small cohort studies.[15]

The nature of MLKIs is also underpinned by substantial heterogeneity with regard to the potential recovery in the typical patient cohort. Despite attempts to establish guidelines, surgical management remains complex and patients rarely return to normal after treatment.[16] Return to work is possible, but it may require workplace or job duty modifications, and only 60% of surgically treated patients generally return to sport.[17] Most studies reporting MLKI treatment outcomes, however, are based on a limited number of subjects and only a few studies have been able to translate high-powered conclusions into eventual outcomes.[17–19]

There is limited information regarding the restoration of knee function during locomotion. Some investigators have described abnormalities in knee kinematics during gait,[20,21] which can lead to unilateral knee joint degeneration.[14] But recognition and correction of gait abnormalities seem necessary for successful long-term outcomes.

This article aims to (1) provide an overview of a large MLKI cohort to identify its specific features, particularly in terms of injury pattern and associated lesions; (2) report their subjective outcomes; and (3) investigate MLKR knee kinematics during locomotion.

INJURY PATTERNS AND DEMOGRAPHIC CHARACTERISTICS
Methods

From the authors' database, all patients treated for MLKI by 3 surgeons, between 1986 and 2017, were identified (**Fig. 1**). The prospective database was created in 2002 dedicated to tracking patient outcomes after MLKR; patients who had MLKI before 2002 were retrospectively added to the database. Patients were either given emergency care primarily or secondarily referred to the authors' center from other institutions.

Inclusion criteria were the following: (1) complete rupture of 2 or more major knee ligaments, such as combined ACL, PCL, MCL, and/or PLC; (2) MLKR performed at the authors' center; and (3) a minimum 1-year follow-up. Patients who had (1) previously injured or undergone surgery on the affected knee, (2) subsequently reinjured the affected knee, or (3) active psychosis/significant mental disability were excluded.

Demographics (gender, age, and body mass index [BMI]), nature of injury (number of ligaments injured and mechanism of injury), and associated injuries (fracture, vascular and nerve injuries, meniscal involvement, and other polytrauma injuries)

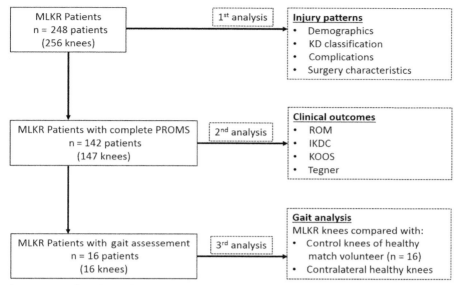

Fig. 1. Study flowchart demonstrating recruitment, to study injury patterns, clinical outcomes, and gait analysis.

were collected. MLKIs were classified according to the modified KDs of the Schenck classification.[22] Treatment details, such as procedure used, timing of surgery, and single or staged procedures, were also reported. Ligamentous reconstruction and/or repair was performed at the discretion of the operating surgeon. Neurovascular status was always assessed before surgery. Any complications and reoperations were registered.

Results

The authors recorded data from 248 consecutives MLKR patients (n = 256 knees). There were 8 bilateral cases, all due to a car or motorbike accident. All patient demographics, characteristics of injury, complications, and main surgery characteristics are reported in **Table 1**.

Demographics
The mean age was 32.5 years ± 13 years (12–73) and the mean BMI was 26.3 ± 4.7 kg/m² (15.8–42.8). There was a predominance of male patients (73%).

Injury mechanisms
The most common mechanisms of injury were road accidents (47%: car 24% and motorbike 23%) followed by sporting injuries (40%), work accidents (2%), falls (1%), and others (10%, nonclassified in the previous categories). Only 1 patient presented a KD related to a with a very low speed mechanism due to obesity.

Injury pattern
According to Schenck classification, there were 29% of KD I (L), 27% of KD I (M), 6% of KD II, 12% of KD III (L), 13% of KD III (M), 4% of KD IV, and 5% of KD V. **Fig. 2** shows the breakdown of injury pattern; a single cruciate combined with a complete lateral or medial injury is the most common.

Table 1
Demographics, injury, and surgery characteristics

Demographics	
Age (mean ±SD [range]) (y)	32.5 ± 12.9 (12–73)
BMI (mean ±SD [range])	26.3 ± 4.7 (15.8–42.8)
Gender: male (%), female (%)	187 (73%), 69 (27%)
Mechanism of injury (%)	
Sport	40.0
Car accident	23.8
Motorbike accident	23.1
Work accident	1.9
Fall	1.3
Others	10.0
Associated lesions (%)	
Meniscal injury	46.1
Medial meniscus injury	25.8
Lateral meniscus injury	31.3
Medial and lateral menisci injury	10.9
Peroneal nerve injury	8.2
Vascular injury	2.7
Timeframe from injury to surgery	
Average timeframe (mean ±SD [range]) (wk)	7 ± 13 (0–54)
Acute (<3 wk) (%)	66
Subacute (3 wk to 3 mo) (%)	19
Chronic (>3 mo) (%)	15
Repair vs reconstruction surgery	
Repair of at least 1 ligament (%) vs reconstruction (%) related to timeframe	
Acute (<3 wk)	47 vs 53
Subacute (3 wk to 3 mo)	30 vs 70
Chronic (>3 mo)	0 vs 100
Repair (%) vs reconstruction (%) related to each ligament	
ACL	3 vs 97
PCL	10 vs 90
LCL-PLC	22 vs 78
MCL-PMC	56 vs 44

Abbreviations: LCL, lateral collateral ligament; PMC, posteromedial corner.

Associated lesions

The overall incidence of common peroneal nerve injury was 8.2%. This complication occurred in 16.7% of lateral or posterolateral injuries, with a higher incidence in KD IL, IIIL, and V stages ($P<.05$). Vascular injury occurred in 2.7% of knees and was present in 5.1% of PCL injuries. No relationship was found between vascular injury and the KD classification. MLKIs were associated with a meniscal injury in 46% of patients; this was most commonly in the lateral meniscus, but 11% of patients sustained a tear of both menisci.

Surgical characteristics

Mean delay to surgery was 7 weeks ± 13 weeks (0–54), with 66% of procedures performed during the acute phase (<3 weeks). The proportion of repair decreased with

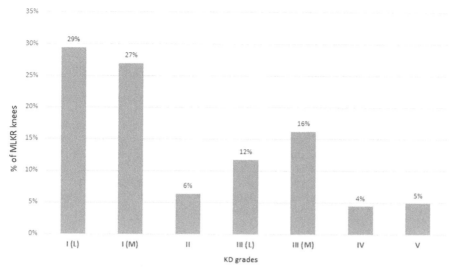

Fig. 2. Percentage breakdown of injury classifications for patients who underwent an MLKR according to the Schenck classification.

the timeframe from injury to surgery. During the acute phase, the proportion of repair of at least 1 ligament was similar to surgery with only reconstruction. After 3 months, surgeries involved only reconstructions. Although cruciate ligaments and PLC were most often reconstructed, the medial side was most often repaired.

Discussion

This study provided information on patterns of patient presentation, injury mechanisms, and treatment approaches, which were similar to those reported in the literature.

With a mean age of 32 years, the authors' study is similar to that reported in the literature, with ages varying between 29 years and 37 years and with an inverse relationship between patient age and risk for MLKI.[15,23] This finding can be explained by the mechanism of injury, which is often associated with high-energy trauma or sports. The authors reported a predominance of male patients, approximately 73%, which is also similar to the 4:1 male-to-female ratio described in most reported MLKI series.[1,15,23] The possible explanation is that male participation is higher in sports that have a risk of collision and a greater risk of knee injury, including MLKI.[24]

With 8.2% of nerve injury and 2.7% of vascular injury, the authors confirmed that neurovascular injuries are frequently associated with an MLKI. In the acute setting of a KD, physicians must carefully evaluate for signs of neurovascular damage. Similarly to Krych and colleagues,[13] the authors also reported that approximately half of the MLKI knees presented a meniscal injury, possibly contributing to the risk of developing early arthrosis.[25]

Regarding the timing of surgery, the literature demonstrated that acute treatment is reported to have better outcomes than delayed treatment.[26,27] Although the authors reported a majority of acute treatment patients, unfortunately, some had been secondarily referred to the authors' center after a delay.

The authors performed repair only in the acute and subacute phases. Primary repairs of bony avulsions, without midsubstance injury, can be done satisfactorily only during the acute phase.[16] After this endpoint, the fibrosis associated with tissue healing makes anatomic reduction and reattachment of injured structures difficult to achieve. Therefore, in injuries older than 3 weeks, it is difficult to achieve primary repair and usually requires a reconstruction.[5,16]

In the authors' study, ligament repair procedure was mostly used for the MCL injury. Management of lateral side injuries is different from that of medial side tears. Medial side injuries are more common than lateral, and a majority can have good outcomes with nonoperative treatment or surgical repair.[28] For the PLC injury, due to an inherent anatomic instability of the lateral tibiofemoral compartment, a reconstruction is often the only solution for a high grade of injury, especially in delayed treatment.[29] Fanelli and colleagues[30] and Levy and colleagues[31] reported a 37% to 40% failure rate with repair compared with 6% to 9% with reconstruction for PLC injury. The authors do note, however, that in their practice, reinforcement of medial repairs with either graft or synthetic material has also become more commonplace in recent times, particularly in the more complex, difficult-to-repair medial side injuries.

CLINICAL OUTCOMES
Methods

From the same cohort, patient-reported outcome measures (PROMs) were assessed via physical examination and functional scores. Objective and subjective scores (International Knee Documentation Committee [IKDC][32] and Knee Injury and Osteoarthritis Outcome Score [KOOS])[33] were assessed at 1 year, 2 years, and at the latest follow-up. Tegner activity level scales[34] were collected before the injury and at the latest follow-up. Only the patients with complete PROMs were included in the analysis (see **Fig. 1**).

Results

A total of 147 patients with complete PROMs were included, at a mean follow-up of 6.1 years $\pm$ 5.5 years.[1,29]

Functional scores
At the last follow-up, the mean IKDC subjective score was 67.23 $\pm$ 20.1 (13.79–100) (**Fig. 3**). For KOOS, daily living (86.78 $\pm$ 13.1 [46–100]) and pain (81.3 $\pm$ 17 [33–100]) subscales improved more than the symptoms (68.5 $\pm$ 16.7 [29–100]), sports (57.4 $\pm$ 29.9 [0–100]), and quality of life (52.7 $\pm$ 25.6 [0–100]) subscales. Before the injury, the median Tegner level was 6. At the last follow-up, Tegner activity levels had a normal distribution, with a median of 5, with a shift of the curves to lower levels of activity compared with preinjury (**Fig. 4**). Therefore, multiligament surgery did not restore the preinjury level of activity ($P<.01$). Whichever of these scores was analyzed, the KD grade did not seem to influence the outcomes ($P>.05$).

Range of motion
At the last follow-up, the mean full flexion was 121.8° $\pm$ 11.8° (90°–145°). Between the injured knee and the contralateral knee, the mean interlimb difference was 7.6°, with 47% of interlimb difference greater than 5°, 31% greater than 10°, and 9% greater than 20°. Although 18 patients displayed an extension deficit greater than or equal to 5° (10%), none had a fixed flexion deformity more than 7°. An interlimb difference greater than 5° was observed for passive extension in 9% of patients.

Discussion

This study represents midterm outcomes of one of the largest series of consecutive MLKIs reported to date. Although there is wide variation in the results, from total

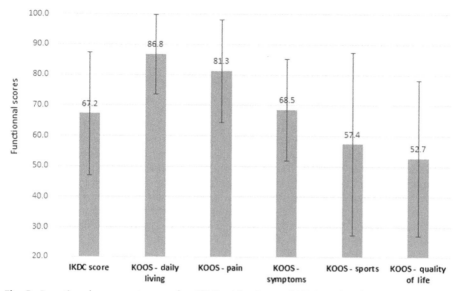

Fig. 3. Functional score outcomes for IKDC subjective and KOOS subscale scores.

disability to nearly full recovery of function, and patient expectations differ from a simple ligament reconstruction due to the complexity of the injury, there are still useful implications from these findings.

Similar to the literature, the authors' outcomes analysis showed that MLKIs have a significant impact on knee function, and patients rarely return to normal after treatment.[35] Compared with a normal population, the functional results of MLKR patients remain low, regardless of the number of injured ligaments or method of treatment.

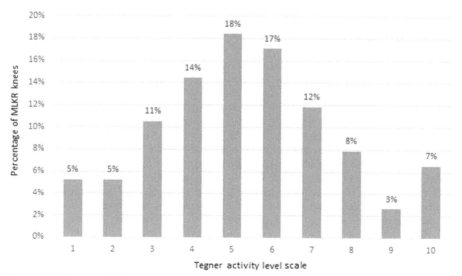

Fig. 4. Distribution of the MLKR knees regarding the Tegner activity level scale at the last follow-up.

After surgery, the overall level of activity is reduced. Restoration of stability and range of motion, however, are usually sufficient to restore normal activities of daily living without pain. In the authors' series, the mean flexion (122° vs 124° for Khakha and colleagues[36]), the mean KOOS activities of daily living subscale (86.78 vs 84 for Khakha and colleagues[36] and 84–91 for Harner and colleagues[37]), and mean Tegner activity level scales (5 vs 4 for Karataglis and colleagues[35]) were similar to the literature.

As concluded by Everhart and colleagues,[17] return to work is frequently possible (88%) after MLKR, although it may require modification of the workplace or job responsibilities (62% with little or no modifications). Similarly, the authors found that 90% of patients could perform light labor and 65% heavy labor tasks after an MLKR. Return to sport, however, occurs in less surgically treated patients. The authors reported that 65% of MLKR patients returnws to sport and only 29% of patients participating in high-level sport could return to the same competitive level. Similarly, the sport subscale of KOOS was one of the most affected at the last follow-up, with a low score of approximately 50. These findings confirm the outcomes reported in the literature, with a return to sport rate of 60% for Everhart and colleagues[17] and 46% to 68% for Stannard and colleagues.[38] Return to a high level of sport has also been reported to be lower (22%).

Some factors have been associated with poor clinical outcomes: nonoperative treatment,[27] delayed surgery,[27] higher injury severity and neurovascular injury,[10,39] obesity,[40] and age greater than 30 years.[41] MLKR with medial or lateral reconstructions demonstrated comparable outcomes.[19,42] As confirmed by Woodmass and colleagues,[3] the functional outcomes after MLKR are primarily influenced by factors other than the knee, including concomitant injuries and psychosocial factors, especially in polytraumatized patients.

GAIT ANALYSIS
Methods

The authors' objective was to determine knee kinematics and gait characteristics of MLKR patients. In this section, the results reported in a previous study are summarized.[20] A subgroup of patients (N = 16; 10 male patients and 6 female patients) were selected from the large cohort described in that study (see Fig. 1). The average time from surgery to gait analysis was 4.7 years ± 3.5 years. MLKR knees were compared with the contralateral knee for each patient and also to matched healthy control knees. Healthy control knees were matched for gender, age, height, and weight (within 10%); were free of any lower limb pathology; and had no prior history of surgery. Both groups underwent 3-D gait analysis. Retroreflective markers were attached to bony landmarks, and their position tracked using a Motion Analysis system during level walking (Motion Analysis, Santa Rosa, California) (Fig. 5). Two force plates (Kistler, Winterthur, Switzerland) were used to record ground reaction forces to identify the heel-strike and toe-off events. Knee kinematics and spatiotemporal gait characteristics were determined using Visual3D v5 (C-Motion, Germantown, Maryland). Interlimb differences in knee angle between each patient's injured limbs, contralateral limbs, and healthy controls were calculated. Coordination strategies between the interacting segments at the lower extremity were quantified using relative phase dynamics. Statistical analyses were performed using single-case (pairwise) and group-aggregated data comparisons.

Results

The group comparison only revealed a few differences, but the single-case analysis detected significant differences for many variables during the subphases of stance,

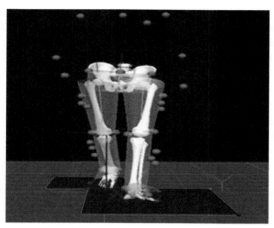

Fig. 5. Model created in visual 3-D used to calculate joint centers and segments.

from heel strike to toe off. Although gait differences are patient-specific, MLKR patients displayed significant alterations in knee kinematics and spatiotemporal gait characteristics not identified in healthy controls during walking.

Knee kinematics

The analysis of the MLKR knee kinematics demonstrated less mobility, with a 25% reduction in average knee flexion during weight acceptance alone, compared with uninjured knees. The pattern of MLKR knee motion was more constrained than that of the healthy knees. The phase coupling of MLKR knees was altered, leading to less coordination between the leg and the thigh.

Gait characteristics

The average velocity of the MLKR patients was significantly reduced compared with the control group ($P<.05$). Patients spent more time in the initial double support phase, with delayed toe off on the reconstructed limb compared with healthy patients ($P<.05$). Single-case analysis revealed other significant differences between both groups. A majority of reconstructed limbs stepped significantly shorter and wider than their matched controls.

Discussion

Gait alterations in MLKR patients are difficult to analyze. In all patient groups, there is high interindividual variability, which when aggregated masks significant individual differences. MLKR patients displayed abnormalities of gait characteristics and of knee kinematics during gait that were not identified in the healthy population.

These differences persisted at 4.7 years after reconstruction and may have important consequences for the knee function. The rigid coordination of the gait pattern[43] associated with a slower gait[44] and shorter steps[45] can lead to an unstable gait with a reduced adaptive capacity and, therefore, an increase in the risk of falling. Finally, as demonstrated by Paterno and Hewett[21] and Hart and colleagues,[14] knee kinematic changes can result in abnormally high stresses on healing tissues, leading to persistent instability and high shearing forces on joint cartilage that result in early osteoarthritis.

Therefore, early diagnosis of gait abnormalities with a specific gait rehabilitation program seems essential for successful long-term outcomes after MLKR. It is clear that this cohort of patients requires an intense, individualized, and longer-term rehabilitation program, with a good understanding of the pathology, to avoid long-term functional deficits and optimize function.

SUMMARY

This study represents midterm outcomes of one of the largest series of consecutive MLKIs reported to date. The present findings highlight road accidents, sporting activities, and male gender as the main risk factors for the presentation of such injuries. The most frequent injury pattern is 1 cruciate ligament tear combined with a complete medial or lateral side injury. Associated lesions, such as neurovascular and meniscal injuries, are frequently combined with MLKI and should always be considered during acute injury assessment. Regardless of the injury severity, the clinical outcomes and the data from gait analysis showed that MLKIs have a significant impact on knee function and patients rarely return to normal after treatment. Future work is required to identify the key modifiable drivers of clinical and gait outcomes in these patients to optimize treatment pathways.

REFERENCES

1. Arom GA, Yeranosian MG, Petrigliano FA, et al. The changing demographics of knee dislocation: a retrospective database review. Clin Orthop 2014;472(9): 2609–14.
2. Johnson ME, Foster L, DeLee JC. Neurologic and vascular injuries associated with knee ligament injuries, neurologic and vascular injuries associated with knee ligament injuries. Am J Sports Med 2008;36(12):2448–62.
3. Woodmass JM, Johnson NR, Mohan R, et al. Poly-traumatic multi-ligament knee injuries: is the knee the limiting factor? Knee Surg Sports Traumatol Arthrosc 2018;26(9):2865–71.
4. Werner BC, Gwathmey FW, Higgins ST, et al. Ultra-low velocity knee dislocations: patient characteristics, complications, and outcomes. Am J Sports Med 2014; 42(2):358–63.
5. Fanelli GC, Orcutt DR, Edson CJ. The multiple-ligament injured knee: evaluation, treatment, and results. Arthroscopy 2005;21(4):471–86.
6. Levy BA, Fanelli GC, Whelan DB, et al. Controversies in the treatment of knee dislocations and multiligament reconstruction. J Am Acad Orthop Surg 2009;17(4): 197–206.
7. Hughston JC, Andrews JR, Cross MJ, et al. Classification of knee ligament instabilities. Part II. The lateral compartment. J Bone Joint Surg Am 1976;58(2):173–9.
8. Alhoukail A, Panu A, Olson J, et al. Intra-articular peroneal nerve incarceration following multi-ligament knee injury. Knee Surg Sports Traumatol Arthrosc 2015; 23(10):3044–8.
9. Werner BC, Norte GE, Hadeed MM, et al. Peroneal nerve dysfunction due to multiligament knee injury: patient characteristics and comparative outcomes after posterior tibial tendon transfer. Clin J Sport Med 2017;27(1):10–9.
10. Sanders TL, Johnson NR, Levy NM, et al. Effect of vascular injury on functional outcome in knees with multi-ligament injury: a matched-cohort analysis. J Bone Joint Surg Am 2017;99(18):1565–71.
11. McDonough EB, Wojtys EM. Multiligamentous injuries of the knee and associated vascular injuries. Am J Sports Med 2009;37(1):156–9.

12. Porrino J, Richardson ML, Hovis K, et al. Association of tibial plateau fracture morphology with ligament disruption in the context of multiligament knee injury. Curr Probl Diagn Radiol 2018;47(6):410–6.
13. Krych AJ, Sousa PL, King AH, et al. Meniscal tears and articular cartilage damage in the dislocated knee. Knee Surg Sports Traumatol Arthrosc 2015;23(10): 3019–25.
14. Hart JM, Blanchard BF, Hart JA, et al. Multiple ligament knee reconstruction clinical follow-up and gait analysis. Knee Surg Sports Traumatol Arthrosc 2009;17(3): 277–85.
15. Wilson SM, Mehta N, Do HT, et al. Epidemiology of multiligament knee reconstruction. Clin Orthop 2014;472(9):2603–8.
16. Moatshe G, Chahla J, LaPrade RF, et al. Diagnosis and treatment of multiligament knee injury: state of the art. J ISAKOS Jt Disord Amp Orthop Sports Med 2017; 2(3):152.
17. Everhart JS, Du A, Chalasani R, et al. Return to work or sport after multiligament knee injury: a systematic review of 21 studies and 524 patients. Arthroscopy 2018;34(5):1708–16.
18. Plancher KD, Siliski J. Long-term functional results and complications in patients with knee dislocations. J Knee Surg 2008;21(4):261–8.
19. Tardy N, Boisrenoult P, Teissier P, et al. Clinical outcomes after multiligament injured knees: medial versus lateral reconstructions. Knee Surg Sports Traumatol Arthrosc 2017;25(2):524–31.
20. Scholes CJ, Lynch JT, Ebrahimi M, et al. Gait adaptations following multiple-ligament knee reconstruction occur with altered knee kinematics during level walking. Knee Surg Sports Traumatol Arthrosc 2017;25(5):1489–99.
21. Paterno MV, Hewett TE. Biomechanics of multi-ligament knee injuries (MLKI) and effects on gait. N Am J Sports Phys Ther 2008;3(4):234–41.
22. Schenck RC. The dislocated knee. Instr Course Lect 1994;43:127–36.
23. Brautigan B, Johnson DL. The epidemiology of knee dislocations. Clin Sports Med 2000;19(3):387–97.
24. de Loës M, Dahlstedt LJ, Thomée R. A 7-year study on risks and costs of knee injuries in male and female youth participants in 12 sports. Scand J Med Sci Sports 2000;10(2):90–7.
25. Badlani JT, Borrero C, Golla S, et al. The effects of meniscus injury on the development of knee osteoarthritis: data from the osteoarthritis initiative. Am J Sports Med 2013;41(6):1238–44.
26. Cook S, Ridley TJ, McCarthy MA, et al. Surgical treatment of multiligament knee injuries. Knee Surg Sports Traumatol Arthrosc 2015;23(10):2983–91.
27. Levy BA, Dajani KA, Whelan DB, et al. Decision making in the multiligament-injured knee: an evidence-based systematic review. Arthroscopy 2009;25(4): 430–8.
28. Laprade RF, Wijdicks CA. The management of injuries to the medial side of the knee. J Orthop Sports Phys Ther 2012;42(3):221–33.
29. LaPrade RF, Resig S, Wentorf F, et al. The effects of grade III posterolateral knee complex injuries on anterior cruciate ligament graft force. A biomechanical analysis. Am J Sports Med 1999;27(4):469–75.
30. Fanelli GC, Stannard JP, Stuart MJ, et al. Management of complex knee ligament injuries. J Bone Joint Surg Am 2010;92(12):2235.
31. Levy BA, Dajani KA, Morgan JA, et al. Repair versus reconstruction of the fibular collateral ligament and posterolateral corner in the multiligament-injured knee. Am J Sports Med 2010;38(4):804–9.

32. Irrgang JJ, Anderson AF, Boland AL, et al. Development and validation of the international knee documentation committee subjective knee form. Am J Sports Med 2001;29(5):600–13.
33. Roos EM, Roos HP, Lohmander LS, et al. Knee Injury and osteoarthritis outcome score (KOOS)–development of a self-administered outcome measure. J Orthop Sports Phys Ther 1998;28(2):88–96.
34. Tegner Y, Lysholm J. Rating systems in the evaluation of knee ligament injuries. Clin Orthop 1985;198:43–9.
35. Karataglis D, Bisbinas I, Green MA, et al. Functional outcome following reconstruction in chronic multiple ligament deficient knees. Knee Surg Sports Traumatol Arthrosc 2006;14(9):843–7.
36. Khakha RS, Day AC, Gibbs J, et al. Acute surgical management of traumatic knee dislocations–Average follow-up of 10 years. Knee 2016;23(2):267–75.
37. Harner CD, Waltrip RL, Bennett CH, et al. Surgical management of knee dislocations. J Bone Joint Surg Am 2004;86-A(2):262–73.
38. Stannard JP, Brown SL, Farris RC, et al. The posterolateral corner of the knee: repair versus reconstruction. Am J Sports Med 2005;33(6):881–8.
39. Hatch GFR, Villacis D, Damodar D, et al. Quality of life and functional outcomes after multiligament knee reconstruction. J Knee Surg 2018;31(10):970–8.
40. Ridley TJ, Cook S, Bollier M, et al. Effect of body mass index on patients with multiligamentous knee injuries. Arthroscopy 2014;30(11):1447–52.
41. Levy NM, Krych AJ, Hevesi M, et al. Does age predict outcome after multiligament knee reconstruction for the dislocated knee? 2- to 22-year follow-up. Knee Surg Sports Traumatol Arthrosc 2015;23(10):3003–7.
42. King AH, Krych AJ, Prince MR, et al. Surgical outcomes of medial versus lateral multiligament-injured, dislocated knees. Arthroscopy 2016;32(9):1814–9.
43. Davids K, Glazier P, Araújo D, et al. Movement systems as dynamical systems: the functional role of variability and its implications for sports medicine. Sports Med 2003;33(4):245–60.
44. Bruijn SM, van Dieën JH, Meijer OG, et al. Is slow walking more stable? J Biomech 2009;42(10):1506–12.
45. Kirkwood RN, de Souza Moreira B, Vallone MLDC, et al. Step length appears to be a strong discriminant gait parameter for elderly females highly concerned about falls: a cross-sectional observational study. Physiotherapy 2011;97(2): 126–31.

Knee Dislocation (KD) IV Injuries of the Knee

Presentation, Treatment, and Outcomes

Dustin L. Richter, MD, Christopher P. Bankhead, MD,
Daniel C. Wascher, MD, Gehron P. Treme, MD,
Andrew Veitch, MD, Robert C. Schenck Jr, MD*

KEYWORDS

- KDIV • Dislocation • Multiligamentous knee injury • MLI

KEY POINTS

- KDIV ligament injuries of the knee are high-energy knee injuries in which both cruciates and both medial and lateral corners are torn.
- KDIV ligament injuries have a higher rate of neurovascular injury than KDIII, II, or I injuries, and have poorer outcomes with respect to return to work as compared with a similar subset of lower-energy KDs.
- KDIV ligament injuries of the knee require treating the patient as a whole, understanding the potential for multitrauma, neurovascular injury, closed head injury, and the determination of management of the ligament injury as an important but oftentimes the last component of care.
- KDIV ligament injuries of the knee may require immediate open exploration due to irreducibility resulting from displaced/locked structures and can present as a posterolateral knee dislocation.
- KDIV ligament injuries of the knee often require closed reduction, temporary external fixation, and delay of ligament reconstructions to provide for patient mobilization and management of soft tissues.

INTRODUCTION

Fundamentally, a knee dislocation (KD) occurs with the disruption of at least 1 cruciate ligament and concurrent loss of reduction of the tibiofemoral articulation. Knee dislocations were once thought to be an extremely rare injury; however, knee dislocations are now being recognized with increasing frequency, particularly in trauma centers. The incidence is increasing because of increased exposure to high-energy trauma,

The authors disclose Educational Grants from Arthrex.
Department of Orthopaedic Surgery, University of New Mexico, MSC10 5600, 1 University of New Mexico, Albuquerque, NM 87131-0001, USA
* Corresponding author.
E-mail address: RSchenck@salud.unm.edu

Clin Sports Med 38 (2019) 247–260
https://doi.org/10.1016/j.csm.2018.11.007
0278-5919/19/© 2018 Elsevier Inc. All rights reserved.

changes in automotive design, and increased recognition of the spontaneously reduced dislocation.[1,2] As this monograph title uses knee MLI (multiligamentous injury of the knee), more than 50% of patients present with a spontaneously reduced knee dislocation.[1] Hence, MLI captures all injuries rather than using the term knee dislocation. Furthermore, spontaneously reduced KDs cannot be classified by the original position classification scheme proposed by Kennedy.[3] It was in such scenarios that the KD or anatomic classification was developed to capture and classify the MLI knee whether spontaneously reduced or dislocated at the time of evaluation.[4]

In the anatomic classification system defined by Schenck[5] and modified by Wascher and colleagues,[1] knee dislocations are classified by the number of ligaments completely disrupted. The different patterns are delineated by roman numerals, with the higher-numbered injuries typically sustaining higher-energy trauma than the lower-numbered patterns (**Table 1**). With the KD system, it is the functional status of ligaments that are used to classify in conjunction with MRI. There are rare instances of injuries involving a single cruciate and an associated collateral ligament with radiographic evidence of dislocation that are classified as KDI. All bicruciate injuries should be considered as knee dislocations. Bicruciate injuries without collateral ligament involvement (KDII) are also uncommon. The most frequent pattern of knee dislocation involves both cruciate ligament and an associated collateral ligament injury (KDIII) accounting for 57.6% to 80.5% of knee dislocations.[6,7] The most severe ligamentous injuries are seen when all 4 major knee ligaments are disrupted (KDIV). In general, the more ligaments injured, the more severe is the knee injury. These KDIV injuries present the orthopedic surgeon with a significant challenge in acute management and in surgical reconstruction of these knees. There is limited high-level evidence on KDIV injuries available to guide treatment decisions, and thus some controversy exists regarding optimal management strategies. This article reviews the evaluation and management of KDIV injuries and reviews treatment guidelines using a basis of 5 case scenarios.

Table 1 Anatomic (Schenck) classification of knee dislocations	
Class	**Injury Description**
KDI	One cruciate torn with subsequent dislocation. Either 1 or both corners torn. KDI implies an intact cruciate ligament in the knee.
KDII	Both cruciates torn with both collaterals intact.
KDIII	Both cruciates torn with 1 corner/collateral torn, subset M or L. KDIIIM if medial side/medial corner torn with both cruciates. KDIIIL if lateral side/lateral corner torn with both cruciates.
KDIV	Both cruciates torn with both collaterals/corners torn.
KDV	Fracture-dislocation of the knee (Wascher modification). *Stannard further described KDVs with following subsets:
KDV-1	Fracture-dislocation with a single cruciate injury.
KDV-2	Fracture-dislocation with both cruciates torn, collaterals/corners intact.
KDV-3	Fracture-dislocation with both cruciates and 1 collateral/corner torn.
KDV-4	Fracture-dislocation with both cruciates and both collaterals/corners torn.

Subscript of C implies arterial injury. Subscript of N implies a nerve injury.
    Example: KDIVCN (patient EG) involves a KDIV with a popliteal artery injury and a peroneal palsy.
    Note: Although initials KD imply "knee dislocation" the anatomic system can be applied to knee dislocations or multiligamentous knee injuries that present spontaneously reduced.
    * Indicates that Dr. Stannard had a further subset of KDV classifications - shown as KDV-1 thru KDV-4.

MECHANISM OF INJURY

Although some knee dislocations are the result of low-energy mechanisms, almost all KDIV injuries are the result of high-energy mechanisms. Typically, these patients are involved in high-speed motor vehicle crashes, pedestrians being struck by vehicles, or falls from a great height.[7,8] Because of the severity of trauma causing these injuries, it is common for these patients to have associated life-threatening injuries to the head, thorax, or abdomen. Likewise, concomitant trauma to the ipsilateral leg or other extremities is common.[1,9,10] Treatment of these associated injuries often takes precedence over the definitive treatment of the knee dislocation and may delay ligament reconstruction; however, it should be remembered that KDIV injuries also can occur in ultra–low-velocity knee dislocations in morbidly obese patients. In the series of Azar colleagues,[11] 5 of 17 patients with ultra–low-velocity dislocations had KDIV injury patterns.

Typically, KDIV injuries are the results of severe rotational trauma, sometimes with associated hyperextension, valgus, or varus forces. The magnitude of the force required to tear all 4 major ligaments also results in significant capsular disruption. These forces also can cause tendon avulsions and neurovascular injuries. Neurovascular injuries occur more commonly in KDIV injuries.[12,13] Stannard and colleagues[13] reported that 16% of KDIV knees had popliteal artery damage. Similarly, common peroneal nerve injuries can result from traction on the nerve as it wraps around the fibular neck.[14,15] Not surprisingly, associated neurovascular injuries have been shown to negatively affect outcomes.[14,16,17]

EVALUATION

When examining a patient with a dislocated knee, the orthopedic surgeon should not forget the basic ABCs of trauma. The orthopedist should participate as needed in resuscitation of the patient's airway, breathing, and circulatory status. Examination for fractures and dislocations in other extremities also should be performed. Once the patient is stabilized, the knee should be examined. It is important to note that the initial physical examination, performed before gross swelling has occurred, is usually the most accurate. The skin about the knee should be examined for open wounds that may communicate with the knee joint and also for abrasions and contusions that may compromise future skin incisions. The knee should be gently ranged and any bony crepitus suggestive of a fracture noted. The extensor mechanism should be palpated, and if possible, tested, to ensure integrity of the patellar tendon. Cruciate ligament laxity should be assessed with the Lachman test (anterior cruciate ligament [ACL]) and posterior drawer (posterior cruciate ligament [PCL]). The collateral ligaments should be subjected to varus and valgus stress at both 30° and at full extension. It is difficult to perform the pivot shift examination on these severely injured knees. Typically, KDIV knees are grossly unstable and care must be taken to ensure that the knee is not left in a dislocated state.

After the ligamentous examination, a careful neurovascular examination should be performed. Light touch sensation of the saphenous, posterior tibia, and the superficial and deep peroneal nerves should be tested. Similarly, motor function of the common peroneal and posterior tibial nerves should be recorded. Krych and colleagues[12] reported that 25.9% of peroneal nerve injuries occur in KDIV injuries. The prognosis is guarded for complete peroneal nerve injuries. Prompt identification of a vascular injury is imperative, as ischemia time of more than 8 hours leads to amputation in up to 86% of patients.[18] A thorough neurovascular examination includes palpation of the dorsalis pedis and posterior tibial pulses and comparing them with the uninjured extremity. It is important to note that limbs with complete loss of flow through the popliteal artery can still present with palpable pulses and a perfused foot from collateral blood flow in the early postinjury period. However, soft tissue swelling will eventually compromise this collateral flow, resulting in an ischemic limb.[19,20]

Stannard and colleagues[13] have described a protocol for selective angiography; the patient is admitted for a minimum of 48 hours and a careful vascular examination is performed at admission, 4 to 6 hours later and then again at 24 and 48 hours after admission. Any pulse abnormality noted before admission or during the serial examination warrants immediate angiography.[13] The Ankle-Brachial Index (ABI) also has been used to identify limbs with potential vascular injury. An ABI less than 0.9 should be followed by an angiogram or duplex ultrasonography to accurately assess the vascular status.[21–23] Because the risk of vascular injury is higher in the KDIV injury, the orthopedic surgeon should have a low threshold for advanced imaging. As these patients are often undergoing computed tomography (CT) scans of other body parts, we will often obtain a CT angiogram of the affected extremity while the patient is in the scanner. Any vascular abnormality on advanced imaging warrants emergent vascular consultation.

Anteroposterior (AP) and lateral radiographs of the knee should be obtained. Radiographs of a dislocated knee in the trauma bay can often reveal avulsion fractures that may be difficult to identify after reduction. However, obtaining radiographs of a dislocated knee should not unduly delay reduction. Reduction of KDIV injuries is usually readily performed with the application of longitudinal traction. A repeat neurovascular examination is mandatory. After reduction, the physician should immobilize the knee in 20° flexion with a locked brace or with splints. Postreduction radiographs should be performed to confirm a satisfactory reduction. An irreducible knee dislocation implies invagination of the capsule and should undergo urgent open reduction in the operative room. Grossly unstable knees require an external fixator to maintain the reduction. In our experience, it is common to apply external fixators to these severe knee injuries. It ensures maintenance of the reduction and facilitates nursing care for the multiply-injured patient.

Advanced imaging techniques should be used in all patients with knee dislocations. If surgery is delayed, varus and valgus stress radiographs can quantitate the amount of collateral ligament laxity. LaPrade and colleagues[24] noted that side-to-side valgus laxity greater than 3.2 mm indicates a complete medial collateral ligament (MCL) tear and Kane and colleagues[25,26] found that a side-to-side varus laxity greater than 2.2 mm or greater than 4.0 mm indicated a complete tear of the lateral collateral ligament (LCL) and posterolateral corner, respectively. CT scan is useful if there is evidence of any bony injury on the plain radiographs. Bony avulsions and subtle distal femur or proximal tibial fractures are best identified with CT scans. MRI should be routinely performed on all suspected knee dislocations. It will confirm the injured cruciate ligaments and also show the location of the collateral ligament tears, which can be useful for surgical planning. Collateral ligament tears near an insertion may be amenable to surgical repair, whereas mid-substance ruptures will necessitate reconstructive techniques. MRI also will reveal meniscal tears, chondral injuries, and tendon avulsions. Combining the initial physical examination with a careful review of the MRI will allow the surgeon to plan definitive treatment of the KDIV injury. A careful examination under anesthesia should be performed at the time of surgery to evaluate the integrity of the ligaments before surgical reconstruction.

TREATMENT GUIDELINES

Once evaluation of the patient has been performed and neurovascular examination is completed, a treatment plan is ready to be developed. Treatment plans may vary based on concomitant injuries, overall health and baseline function, and ability to participate in an aggressive postsurgical rehabilitation protocol. KDIVs frequently require external fixation, but when presenting in an isolated fashion can be repaired or reconstructed in one setting. Definitive management can vary from brace immobilization or external fixation to acute or delayed repair or reconstruction.[27–29] The authors present an overall description and guidelines for 4 basic presentations of a KDIV injury, with an additional fifth case that required a staged revision reconstruction and posterior tibial tendon transfer performed before reconstruction.

CASE 1: Poly-trauma patient with a closed head injury → KDIV requiring initial external fixation with delayed ligamentous reconstruction

24-year-old woman (CJ) who was the helmeted driver of a motorcycle that lost control and crashed. Trauma workup demonstrated a subarachnoid hemorrhage, splenic laceration with active bleeding, nondisplaced pelvic fracture, and dislocated left knee classified as a KDIV. She was taken emergently to the operating room by general surgery for laparotomy, and orthopedics was consulted. She was noted to have a left knee dislocation (**Fig. 1**A) that was reducible. Distal pulses were palpable and ABIs were symmetric bilaterally. Examination at that time under anesthesia revealed a KDIV injury pattern. The knee was reduced and placed into a knee immobilizer with serial vascular examinations.

MRI confirmed the KDIV injury (**Fig. 1**B, C). The patient's poly-trauma and head injury required intubation and sedation. The patient's knee reduction could not be maintained with bracing and with her closed head injury preventing participation in a rehabilitation program, application of a knee spanning external fixator was necessary (**Fig. 1**D). The patient was hospitalized in the intensive care unit/trauma unit for approximately 1 month. The patient gradually improved from her head injury and became conversant, was able to care for herself and participate in physical therapy. The external fixator was removed after 7 weeks with concomitant manipulation under anesthesia demonstrating full range of motion (ROM) but laxity in all planes consistent with a KDIV injury and no significant interval ligamentous healing.

The patient underwent definitive 4-ligament allograft reconstruction 6 months after initial injury (**Fig. 1**E–H). Deep vein thrombosis (DVT) prophylaxis was used with low-dose aspirin for a total of 6 weeks. She regained full ROM with excellent stability and was living and working independently 3 months out from surgery, with final follow-up at 5 years. There was evidence of heterotopic ossification noted in the region of the proximal MCL as a result of the knee injury and in all likelihood accentuated by her closed head injury.

CASE 2: Isolated irreducible KDIV → Semi-emergent open reduction and repair/reconstruction

43-year-old man (TA), active duty military, sustained a crash while snowboarding in a ski resort 4 hours away from the level I trauma center. Initially seen at outside facility, where he was noted to have both a right knee tibiofemoral and patella dislocation. This was an isolated injury. Reduction was attempted twice unsuccessfully at the outside facility and the patient transferred for additional care.

On arrival to the tertiary care hospital, persistent tibiofemoral subluxation with patella dislocation was noted. Partial reduction was performed and placed into a brace. CT angiogram was performed demonstrating an intact popliteal artery and distal vasculature. He had an MRI performed demonstrating the KDIV injury with a peel-off PCL tear, medial patellofemoral ligament avulsion, and locked medial and lateral meniscus tears with tibiofemoral subluxation. Interestingly,

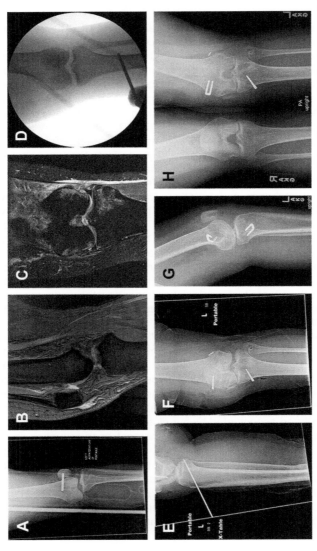

Fig. 1. (*A*) Complete dislocation of the knee. Note the AP appearance of the femur and lateral of the tibia. (*B, C*) Selective cuts of the MR with bone bruising, KDIV involvement. MR can be extremely useful for documenting the integrity of the extensor mechanism in such high-energy injuries. (*D*) AP radiograph of the knee after external fixation. (*E–H*) Intraoperative and long-term radiographs for simultaneous 4-ligament knee reconstruction using allografts. We currently avoid staples to prevent painful implants.

the patient also had a tear of an accessory head of the gastrocnemius with entrapment in the knee joint. On return from advanced imaging, the brace had been loosened and the patient again required repeat reduction, given the profound instability in the knee (**Fig. 2**A, B).

The patient was diagnosed as having a complex or irreducible knee dislocation (posterolateral knee dislocation with medial knee skin furrowing) and operative open reduction was planned. External fixation would not be indicated in this patient, as it was irreducible and carries the added risk of medial soft tissue necrosis from the medial furrowing and displacement. The patient was taken to the operating room and a brief arthroscopy was performed followed by open reduction of the medial structures, repair of the medial and lateral menisci, removal of the medial gastrocnemius from the knee joint, repair of the PCL peel-off lesion, ACL and MCL reconstruction, and repair of the large avulsion of the posterolateral corner (**Fig. 2**C, D). DVT prophylaxis was used with initial injectable short-chain heparin followed by low-dose aspirin for a total of 6 weeks. Postoperatively, the patient did well. He was able to play soccer with his kids, perform box jumps, and pass the military running requirement. He did most activities in a knee brace without any frank instability. He returned to snowboarding using a brace.

CASE 3: Isolated, neurovascularly intact KDIV → 4-ligament arthroscopic-assisted reconstruction after regaining motion

32-year-old man (RB) involved in a motor vehicle collision outside of the state and sustained an isolated left knee MLI presenting reduced at time of evaluation but classified as a KDIV. He was admitted to the outside hospital for several days and then discharged in a knee brace. He presented for knee instability, pain, and stiffness 2 months postinjury with ROM from 2° of a flexion contracture to 95° of knee flexion. The patient had difficulty bearing weight and had to use crutches to ambulate. Despite his flexion loss, the patient had gross instability on clinical examination as a KDIV, with advanced imaging consistent with that diagnosis (**Fig. 3**A–D).

Given the limitations in motion, persistent pain, and trouble weightbearing 2 months out from injury, the patient underwent an intra-articular cortisone injection and aggressive physical therapy. The patient returned in 6 weeks with improvement in gait, ROM from 0 to 130° of flexion, but persistent instability. The patient was able to perform a straight leg raise and walk with a heel-to-toe gait. Stress radiographs were obtained to confirm medial and lateral joint opening with both valgus and varus stress, respectively (**Fig. 3**E, F).

The patient underwent an arthroscopic-assisted ACL reconstruction with allograft, PCL reconstruction with allograft via a tibial inlay approach, and open MCL and PLC reconstruction with allograft (**Fig. 3**G, H). Intraoperatively, the bicruciate reconstruction was performed first, followed by the MCL/PMC and then a lateral approach with the posterolateral LaPrade[30] reconstruction. Postoperatively he was kept non-weightbearing for 6 weeks but was allowed early ROM in a brace to avoid recurrence of his preoperative stiffness. DVT prophylaxis was used with low-dose aspirin for a total of 6 weeks. The patient healed well with good stability and ambulated without any assistive devices by 8 weeks. He returned to work, exercise at the gym, and recreational activities. He eventually developed some painful hardware that was removed 3 years out from the index procedure. He currently is 3.5 years out from reconstruction with maintained good stability.

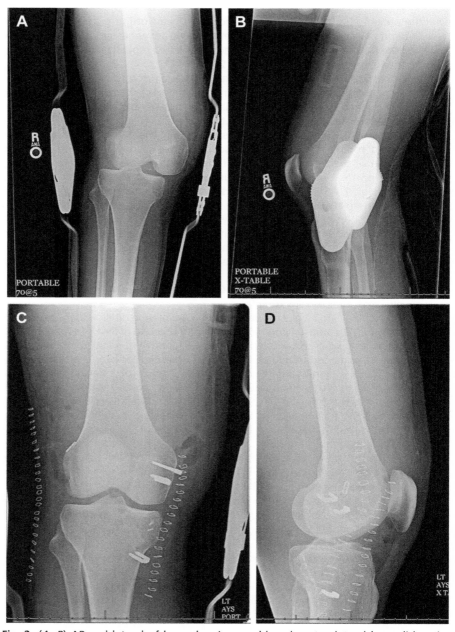

Fig. 2. (*A, B*) AP and lateral of knee showing a subluxed posterolateral knee dislocation requiring immediate open reduction and repair. (*C, D*) Postoperative AP and lateral radiograph after immediate repair/reconstruction.

CASE 4: Chronic KDIV with varus alignment and varus thrust → Staged reconstruction with initial medial opening wedge osteotomy

43-year-old woman (DD) presented to clinic with chronic right knee multiligament injury from a motor vehicle collision 10 years prior. Was treated nonoperatively

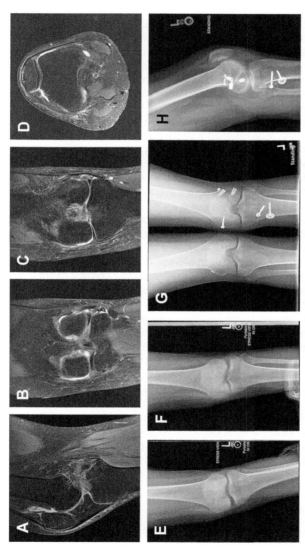

Fig. 3. (A–D) Selective MR cuts of the knee MLI presenting with stiffness and gross instability as a KDIV. (E, F) Stress radiographs showing involvement of both corners. Stress radiographs are extremely valuable in determining ligamentous involvement of the corners in the setting of profound multiligamentous instability. (G, H) Postoperative radiographs of patient after a simultaneous 4-ligament reconstruction.

at an outside facility with extensive physical therapy, medications including cortisone and hyaluronic acid injections, and bracing. Primary concerns were both medial-sided knee pain and gross instability.

The gross ligamentous instability was documented as a KDIV on clinical imaging, radiographic imaging, and MRI. Patient ambulated with a varus thrust and full-length hip-to-ankle weightbearing alignment images revealed 4° of varus (**Fig. 4**A) and a staged osteotomy was performed to create a neutral axis (**Fig. 4**B, C). Because the patient had a concomitant ACL and PCL, the posterior slope was not changed during the osteotomy. DVT prophylaxis was used with initial injectable short-chain heparin followed by low-dose aspirin for a total of 6 weeks. Although it is possible with the osteotomy alone that the patient may have alleviation of her pain and some of her instability symptoms, stage 2 four-ligament reconstruction is planned once the osteotomy heals.

CASE 5: KDIVCN with failed primary reconstruction → Posterior tibial tendon transfer and bone grafting with staged 4-ligament reconstruction

33-year-old woman (EG) referred 5 years out from the index procedure treating a right KDIVCN injury at an outside institution. The patient had suffered a popliteal injury and peroneal nerve palsy following a motorcycle crash 7 years prior. The patient underwent 3 consecutive surgeries with a popliteal artery repair, followed by a 3-ligament knee reconstruction of her KDIV injury (MCL was not reconstructed), and eventual arthroscopy for a medial meniscus tear (**Fig. 5**A, B).

The patient presented to our service with continued instability, a steppage gait, and was initially fitted for an ankle foot orthosis (AFO). The patient desired knee stability but was equally bothered by her foot drop and desired an ability to get out of an AFO. Preoperative duplex arterial and venous ultrasonography revealed a clotted popliteal artery graft and no evidence of DVT. Vascular surgery was consulted and arterial flow was deemed adequate for reconstruction purposes with the use of a tourniquet.

The patient underwent staged procedures with knee hardware removal, tunnel grafting with allograft bone chips and bone marrow aspirate concentrate with simultaneous posterior tibial tendon transfer, and Achilles tendon lengthening. Foot drop and equinus contracture can potentially cause more disability and functional limitations than a knee MLI. Furthermore, delaying posterior tibial tendon transfer can make knee rehabilitation difficult for the patient.[16]

Three months after transfer and grafting, the patient ambulated without an AFO and then underwent 4-ligament knee reconstruction (**Fig. 5**C, D). DVT prophylaxis was used with initial injectable short-chain heparin followed by low-dose aspirin for a total of 6 weeks for both procedures. The patient ambulated brace-free without instability at 3-year follow-up.

CLINICAL OUTCOMES

Overall there is limited high-level evidence on KDIV injuries available to guide treatment decisions. Many studies have excluded these severe KDIV and KDV injuries from their analyses, whereas other outcome studies are not appropriately powered to infer any clinical implications due to the small number of subjects. As a result of the scarcity of knee MLI, lack of consensus on ideal clinical management of this injury, and nonstandardized reporting of outcomes following treatment of knee MLI, clinical outcome studies are limited primarily to case series with varying treatment protocols and outcome measures.

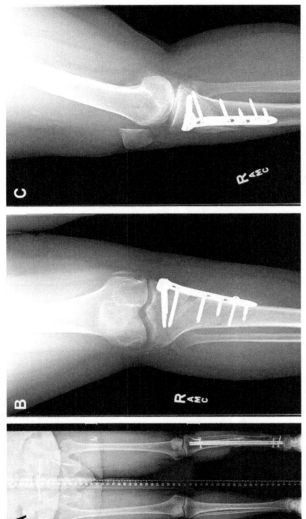

Fig. 4. (A) Full-length hip-to-ankle weightbearing alignment radiograph revealing 4° of varus. (B, C) Immediate postoperative radiographs following a staged proximal tibia medial opening wedge osteotomy to create a neutral axis.

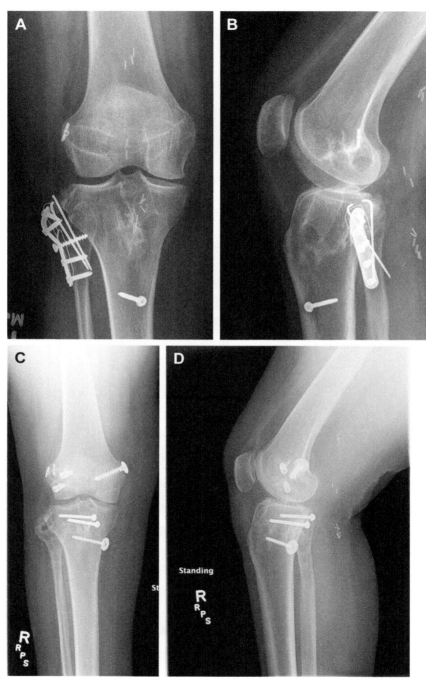

Fig. 5. (*A*, *B*) Preoperative AP and lateral radiographs demonstrating prior ACL, PCL, and posterolateral corner reconstruction with subsequent clinical failure. (*C*, *D*) AP and lateral radiographs following the stage 2 reconstruction after prior hardware removal and bone grafting.

Outcomes have been reported on KDIV patients recently in 2018 that revealed a poor prognosis as compared with KDI, II, and III injuries. In one recent meta-analysis, patients with KDIV had a lower return to work and return to sport than KDIII injuries.[8] This finding is in all likelihood multifactorial with the severity of injury to the knee but also with the potential for associated injuries seen with multitrauma patients. Cook and colleagues[31] found that patients with dislocations with 4-ligament injury were more likely to undergo revision surgery for persistent instability.

SUMMARY

KDIV multiligamentous injuries are complex and significantly devastating injuries to the knee. The approach to such injury patterns is dependent on patient presentation, obesity, poly-trauma, and ability to participate in rehabilitation. If seen in isolation, a standard approach for ligamentous reconstruction can be used but is dependent on chronicity. We used 5 patients to demonstrate a standardized approach to the KDIV with eventual ligamentous reconstruction of all 4 ligaments. Management of knee position is often required with an external fixator, as seen with closed head injury, arterial injury and popliteal artery reconstruction, multitrauma, or obesity. Staged removal of the external fixator, manipulation under anesthesia, and evaluation of ligamentous healing will determine eventual knee ligament reconstruction. Experience and preference often determine the timing of ligament reconstruction and, usually, cruciates are reconstructed first followed by the medial then lateral corners. We prefer to limit our tourniquet time to 2 hours, and anticoagulate patients postoperatively for 6 weeks until weightbearing fully. There is a need for further outcomes studies of knee MLIs with large patient numbers to identify appropriate surgical timing, including the use of early or late reconstruction and repair, which is the topic of one recent multicenter trial.

REFERENCES

1. Wascher DC, Dvirnak PC, DeCoster TA. Knee dislocation: initial assessment and implications for treatment. J Orthop Trauma 1997;11:525–9.
2. Meyers M, Harvey JP. Traumatic dislocation of the knee joint. J Bone Joint Surg Am 1971;53:16–29.
3. Kennedy JC. Complete dislocation of the knee joint. J Bone Joint Surg Am 1963; 45:889–904.
4. Walker DN, Hardison RR, Schenck RC Jr. A baker's dozen of knee dislocations. Am J Knee Surg 1994;7:117–24.
5. Schenck RC Jr. The dislocated knee. Instr Course Lect 1994;43:127–36.
6. Levy NM, Krych AJ, Hevesi M, et al. Does age predict outcome after multiligament knee reconstruction for the dislocated knee? 2- to 22-year follow-up. Knee Surg Sports Traumatol Arthrosc 2015;23:3003–7.
7. Moatshe G, Dornan GJ, Loken S, et al. Demographics and injuries associated with knee dislocation: a prospective review of 303 patients. Orthop J Sports Med 2017;5(5). 2325967117706521.
8. Everhart JS, Du A, Chalasani R, et al. Return to work or sport after multiligament knee injury: a systematic review of 21 studies and 524 patients. Arthroscopy 2018;1:1–9.
9. Lustig S, Leray E, Boisrenoult P, et al. Dislocation and bicruciate lesions of the knee: epidemiology and acute stage assessment in a prospective series. Orthop Traumatol Surg Res 2009;95:614–20.

10. Becker EH, Watson JD, Dreese JC. Investigation of multiligamentous knee injury patterns with associated injuries presenting at a level 1 trauma center. J Orthop Trauma 2013;27:226–31.

11. Azar FM, Brandt JC, Miller RH 3rd, et al. Ultra-low-velocity knee dislocations. Am J Sports Med 2011;39:2170–4.

12. Krych AJ, Giuseffi SA, Kuzma SA, et al. Is peroneal nerve injury associated with worse function after knee dislocation? Clin Orthop Relat Res 2014;472:2630–6.

13. Stannard JP, Sheils TM, Lopez-Ben RR, et al. Vascular injuries in knee dislocations: the role of physical examination in determining the need for arteriography. J Bone Joint Surg Am 2004;86:910–5.

14. Johnson ME, Foster L, DeLee JC. Neurologic and vascular injuries associated with knee ligament injuries. Am J Sports Med 2008;36:2448–62.

15. LaPrade RF, Terry GC. Injuries to the posterolateral aspect of the knee: association of anatomic injury patterns with clinical instability. Am J Sports Med 1997;25:433–8.

16. Peskun CJ, Chahal J, Steinfeld ZY, et al. Risk factors for peroneal nerve injury and recovery in knee dislocation. Clin Orthop Relat Res 2012;470:774–8.

17. Cush G, Irgit K. Drop foot after knee dislocation: evaluation and treatment. Sports Med Arthrosc Rev 2011;19:139–46.

18. Green NE, Allen BL. Vascular injuries associated with dislocation of the knee. J Bone Joint Surg Am 1977;59:236–9.

19. Treiman BC, Yellin AE, Weaver FA, et al. Examination the patient with a knee dislocation: the case for selective arteriography. Arch Surg 1992;127:1056–63.

20. Wascher DC. High-velocity knee dislocation with vascular injury: treatment principles. Clin Sports Med 2000;19:457–77.

21. Mills WJ, Barei DP, McNair P. The value of the ankle-brachial index for diagnosing arterial injury after knee dislocation: a prospective study. J Trauma 2004;56:1261–5.

22. Tocci SL, Heard WM, Fadale PD, et al. Magnetic resonance angiography for the evaluation of vascular injury in knee dislocations. J Knee Surg 2010;23:201–7.

23. Abou-Sayed H, Berger DL. Blunt lower-extremity trauma and popliteal artery injuries: revisiting the case for selective arteriography. Arch Surg 2002;137:585–9.

24. LaPrade RF, Bernhardson AS, Griffith CJ, et al. Correlation of valgus stress radiographs with medial knee ligament injuries: an in vitro biomechanical study. Am J Sports Med 2010;38:330–8.

25. Kane PW, Cinque ME, Moatshe G, et al. Fibular collateral ligament: varus stress radiographic analysis using 3 different clinical techniques. Orthop J Sports Med 2018;6(5):1–6.

26. LaPrade RF, Heikes C, Bakker AJ, et al. The reproducibility and repeatability of varus stress radiographs in the assessment of isolated fibular collateral ligament and grade-III posterolateral knee injuries: an in vitro biomechanical study. J Bone Joint Surg Am 2008;90:2069–76.

27. Rihn JA, Groff YJ, Harner CD, et al. The acutely dislocated knee: evaluation and management. J Am Acad Orthop Surg 2004;12:334–46.

28. Montgomery TJ, Savoie FH, White JL, et al. Orthopedic management of knee dislocations: comparison of surgical reconstruction and immobilization. Am J Knee Surg 1995;8:97–103.

29. Levy BA, Dajani KA, Whelan DB. Decision making in the multiligament-injured knee: an evidence-based systemic review. Arthroscopy 2009;25:430–8.

30. Cruz RS, Mitchell JJ, Dean CS, et al. Anatomic posterolateral corner reconstruction. Arthrosc Tech 2016;5(3):e563–72.

31. Cook S, Ridley TJ, McCarthy MA, et al. Surgical treatment of multiligament knee injuries. Knee Surg Sports Traumatol Arthrosc 2015;23:2983–91.

Fibular Collateral Ligament/ Posterolateral Corner Injury

When to Repair, Reconstruct, or Both

Mitchell I. Kennedy, BS[a], Andrew Bernhardson, MD[b],
Gilbert Moatshe, MD, PhD[c,d], Patrick S. Buckley, MD[b],
Lars Engebretsen, MD, PhD[c,d], Robert F. LaPrade, MD, PhD[b,e,f],*

KEYWORDS

- Posterolateral corner • Anatomic reconstruction • Multiligament injury

KEY POINTS

- Posterolateral corner (PLC) injuries rarely occur in isolation.
- There is a higher risk of concomitant peroneal nerve and vascular injuries in multiligament injuries with PLC injuries.
- Repair of the PLC structures has high (up to 40%) failure rates.
- Reconstruction of the PLC leads to improved patient outcomes and has low failure rates.

INTRODUCTION

The 3 main stabilizing structures of the posterolateral corner (PLC) are the fibular (lateral) collateral ligament (FCL), the popliteus tendon (PLT), and the popliteofibular ligament (PFL). These structures are the primary knee stabilizers that resist varus and external tibial rotation forces. Historically, injuries to the PLC were treated nonoperatively, often leading to persistent instability, poor patient outcomes, and the development of early osteoarthritis. Limited knowledge of the anatomy and biomechanics, coupled with poor patient outcomes with nonoperative management, resulted in the PLC often labeled as the "dark side" of the knee. Currently, grade III PLC injuries are treated surgically. Both surgical repair and reconstruction have been

[a] Steadman Philippon Research Institute, Vail, CO 81657, USA; [b] The Steadman Clinic, 181 West Meadow Drive, Vail, CO 81657, USA; [c] Oslo University Hospital, University of Oslo, PO Box 4950 Nydalen, N-0424, Oslo, Norway; [d] OSTRC, Norwegian School of Sport Sciences, Postboks 4014 Ullevål stadion, Oslo 0806, Norway; [e] Complex Knee and Sports Medicine Surgery, Orthopaedic Surgery, University of Minnesota, Minneapolis, MN, USA; [f] College of Veterinary Medicine and Biomedical Sciences, Colorado State University, Fort Collins, CO, USA
* Corresponding author. The Steadman Clinic, 181 West Meadow Drive, Suite 400, Vail, CO 81657.
E-mail address: laprademdphd@gmail.com

Clin Sports Med 38 (2019) 261–274
https://doi.org/10.1016/j.csm.2018.11.002
0278-5919/19/© 2018 Elsevier Inc. All rights reserved.

sportsmed.theclinics.com

demonstrated to be superior to nonoperative treatment; however, studies comparing reconstruction to repair have reported higher failure rates with surgical repair. In recent years, there have been studies that have elucidated a better understanding of the PLC and led to development of anatomic reconstructions that have resulted in improved patient outcomes. The anatomy and biomechanics of the PLC, a biomechanically validated anatomic PLC reconstruction, and treatment rationale for PLC injuries are discussed.

KEY STRUCTURES—ANATOMY AND BIOMECHANICS

The 3 primary stabilizing structures of the PLC are the FCL, the PLT, and PFL (**Fig. 1**).

Fibular (Lateral) Collateral Ligament

The FCL attaches 1.4-mm proximal and 3.1-mm posterior to the lateral femoral epicondyle and inserts 8.2-mm posterior to the anterior margin of the fibular head and 28.4-mm distal to the apex of the fibular styloid process, with an approximate length of 69.6 mm (**Fig. 2**).[1] The femoral attachment has a cross-sectional area of 0.48 cm^2 and is located in a small bony depression, with additional fanlike fibers extending proximally and anteriorly over the lateral epicondyle.[1] On the fibular head the cross-sectional area of the FCL attachment is 0.43 cm^2 and it is located at 38% of the width of the fibular head. The FCL acts as the primary varus stabilizer of the knee,[2–5] while also providing restraint to tibial external rotation up to 30° of knee flexion,[6] and it also acts as a secondary stabilizer to internal rotation.[7]

A   **B**

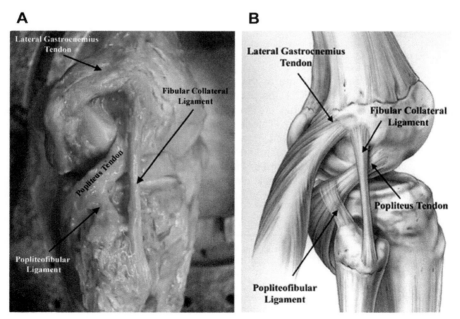

Fig. 1. Lateral view photograph (*A*) and illustration (*B*) of an anatomic identification of the FCL, PLT, PFL, and lateral gastrocnemius tendon on a right knee. (*From* LaPrade RF, Ly TV, Wentorf FA, et al. The posterolateral attachments of the knee: a qualitative and quantitative morphologic analysis of the fibular collateral ligament, popliteus tendon, popliteofibular ligament, and lateral gastrocnemius tendon. Am J Sports Med 2003;31:856; with permission.)

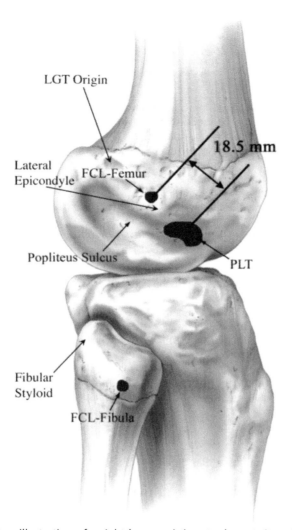

Fig. 2. Lateral view illustration of a right knee and the attachment sites of the PLT in the popliteus sulcus of the femur and the FCL on the femur and fibula. PLT, popliteus tendon. (*From* LaPrade RF, Ly TV, Wentorf FA, et al. The posterolateral attachments of the knee: a qualitative and quantitative morphologic analysis of the fibular collateral ligament, popliteus tendon, popliteofibular ligament, and lateral gastrocnemius tendon. Am J Sports Med 2003;31:857; with permission.)

Popliteus Tendon

The PLT is a structure forming from the proximal third of the popliteal fossa of the popliteus muscle, which courses proximally and laterally from its attachment on the posteromedial tibia.[1] On conversion to tendinous tissue, the PLT becomes intra-articular and courses anterolaterally around the posterior aspect of the lateral femoral condyle, just medial to the FCL, and attaches on the proximal fifth of the popliteal sulcus, anterior to the FCL attachment (see **Fig. 2**). The PLT also functions as a ligament, mainly by functioning as a stabilizer for external rotation in the knee,[7,8] while also providing secondary stabilization of varus stress[8,9]; another feature of the PLT includes minor contributions to anteroposterior tibial translation (specifically in full extension or deficiency of either cruciate ligament).[2,8,10]

Popliteofibular Ligament

The PFL, historically called the arcuate ligament, originates from the musculotendinous junction of the popliteus, becoming 2 divisions, anterior and posterior, with the posterior division always larger than the former.[1] The anterior and posterior division both attach to the popliteus complex at the proximolateral musculotendinous junction, but the anterior division attaches distolaterally on the anterior downslope of the medial aspect of the fibular styloid process, 2.8-mm distal to the tip of the fibular styloid, whereas the posterior division attaches at the apex of the fibular styloid process, less distal to the apex of the fibular styloid process (see **Fig. 2**).[1] The anterior division additionally has fibers extending to the lateral tibia in close proximity to the proximal anterior tibiofibular ligament.[1] The PFL acts as a secondary varus and internal rotation stabilizer.

INJURY MECHANISM

The mechanism of injury to the PLC usually involves direct varus stress, contact or noncontact hyperextension, or twisting of the knee. Only 28% of the PLC injuries occur in isolation and are typically associated with anterior cruciate ligament (ACL) or posterior cruciate ligament (PCL) tears.[11,12] Other concomitant injuries to the structures of the PLC of the knee, including fibular head fractures, biceps femoris tendon avulsions, lateral capsular and iliotibial band avulsions off bone, and common peroneal nerve injuries, have been reported. Furthermore, in the setting of knee dislocations, PLC injuries have been associated with concomitant common peroneal nerve and popliteal artery injuries.[13]

SURGICAL TREATMENT

The PLC was historically considered the dark side of the knee due to a lack of understanding of its anatomy, function, and optimal treatment. In recent years, studies have elucidated the anatomy and biomechanics of the PLC structures. This has led to the development of anatomically based and biomechanically validated PLC reconstruction techniques. Several nonanatomic reconstructions have been reported; however, there is growing interest in and clinical data supporting anatomic reconstruction of torn knee ligaments.

Nonoperative Management

Grade I and grade II PLC injuries are considered partial tears and are defined as a mild (1+) or moderate (2+) varus instability of the knee examined at 30° knee flexion, with full stability in extension, whereas grade III tears display severe (3+) varus translation at 30° and mild or moderate instability in extension.[14] Nonoperative treatment is usually recommended for patients with grade 1 or grade 2 sprains because they lack chronic ligament insufficiency, with follow-up scores showing positive results of return of activity level and radiographic evaluation displaying little to no evidence of posttraumatic osteoarthritis.[14] Nonoperative management of grade III injuries, however, not only display persistent lateral instability but also commonly include anterior and anterolateral instability.[14] In addition to these results, studies have demonstrated that grade III PLC injuries do not heal when treated nonoperatively, due to the bony anatomy of 2 opposing convex surfaces present in the lateral compartment of the knee in humans. Therefore, surgical management is recommended to restore knee stability in grade III PLC injuries.[15–17]

Repair Versus Reconstruction Techniques

The decision to repair or reconstruct the main structures of the PLC in grade III injuries has been debated in the literature. In general, repair of the PLC focuses primarily on reattachment of the FCL and other important structures to their anatomic locations using suture anchors after decortication of bone at the insertion points. Reconstruction aims to use autogenous or allograft tendons placed through bone tunnels at the appropriate anatomic attachment sites and secured with interference screws. Based on lower reported failure rates with PLC reconstruction, however, the pendulum has swung favoring PLC reconstruction in most patient situations.

Multiple reconstruction techniques have been described. Early in the literature, Stannard and colleagues[18] described a reconstruction technique that focused on placing the PLC reconstruction grafts at the anatomic attachments of the major structures of the PLC (PLT, PFL, and FCL) by a modified 2-tailed technique while also using concurrent repair of avulsions in acute injuries. The performed technique uses the isometric point on the femur, a point superior to where the FCL and popliteus cross one another at the lateral femoral condyle.[1] Isolated FCL injuries were reconstructed by femoral fixation with a metal interference screw at the FCL attachment site that was identified relative to both anatomic[1] and radiographic landmarks[19]; a bioabsorbable interference screw is then used for the fibular attachment of the FCL.

Stannard and colleagues[18] used the 2-tailed technique for complete PLC reconstructions relative to repairs and reported failure rates of the repair cohort (37%) significantly higher than the reconstruction cohort (9%). Similar results were reported by Levy and colleagues,[20] when comparing the reconstruction versus repair of FCL tears; they found an overall failure rate of 40% for the repair cohort and 6% for the reconstruction cohort.

Acute Posterolateral Corner Treatment

Geeslin and LaPrade[21] detailed how a combination of both repair and reconstruction techniques can be an effective means for treatment of acutely injured PLC structures depending on the situation of how the structures become injured. Patients with grade III PLC knee injuries who presented in the acute setting (average 17 days from injury) were treated with repair of avulsion fractures, as long as there was no notion that the structure had stretched during the injury mechanism and the anatomic attachment could be reduced with the knee in full extension. Primary repair was optimal during the acute phase because the individual anatomic components were most easily identifiable earlier after injury[22,23] and the ability of injured structures to hold sutures decreases as time between injury and treatment increases and tissue remodeling occurs.[24] The PFL could receive a direct repair only if the PLT was intact and sufficient tissue was present for reapproximation by suturing.[12] Femoral avulsions of the PLT were repaired using the recess procedure, in which an eyelet pin was drilled from the attachment site of the PLT[1] anteromedially across the femur, followed by reaming of a 5-mm diameter tunnel to 1-cm depth.[21] The whipstitched end of the PLT is then pulled into the tunnel and the sutures are tied over a button with the knee in full extension.

The PFL was also repaired using a suture anchor, but in cases where a repair could not be managed with a concurrent FCL reconstruction, the PFL underwent reconstruction. Reconstruction then occurred by looping the portion of the FCL graft that passes out of the posteromedial aspect of the fibular head tunnel around the intact PLT at the musculotendinous junction and passed back laterally, where it was sutured onto itself.

Any structural damage of the 3 main PLC static stabilizers occurring by means other than avulsion, including midsubstance tears, were treated by reconstruction. Anatomic PLC reconstruction (discussed later) of the FCL or PLT was performed using an autogenous hamstring graft,[8,25] unless both structures were torn, in which case the reconstruction was performed with an Achilles tendon allograft.[26,27]

Patients were able to retain objective knee stability from this treatment protocol determined by significantly improved International Knee Documentation Committee and Cincinnati Knee Rating System subjective scores relative to prior reported chronic PLC injuries.[26] A majority of acute PLC repairs in the literature have been documented with good or fair outcomes,[22,23,28] whereas repairs outside of the acute setting have been reported with failure rates as high as 37%[18] to 40%,[20] which is why PLC repair should be used exclusively in acute settings, with PLC reconstruction favorable outside of the 3-week postinjury time period.

Chronic Posterolateral Corner Treatment

Additional patient factors need to be considered when examining the patient with a chronic PLC injury. Most importantly, mechanical axis alignment should be examined with weight-bearing hip-knee-ankle radiographs. For chronic PLC injuries with concurrent genu varus alignment, resolving the mechanical axis malalignment with a biplanar osteotomy has become the accepted protocol prior to PLC reconstruction to prevent future complications with the reconstruction.[29,30] Arthur and colleagues[31] conducted a prospective study assessing chronic PLC deficiency and genu varus alignment treated by proximal tibial opening wedge osteotomy and found that one-third of the patients did not require the second stage PLC reconstruction after a sufficient healing period and rehabilitation protocol.

When addressing chronic or nonavulsion injuries to structures of the PLC, reconstruction is recommended. Positive outcomes have resulted from reconstruction procedures in the literature, corroborated by a systematic review conducted by Geeslin and colleagues,[32] which found that chronic PLC injuries surgically managed with reconstruction procedures have a 90% success rate and 10% failure rate. The surgical techniques used included fibular slings,[33–37] isometric reconstructions,[38–41] and anatomic-based techniques[26] (these reconstruction procedures are displayed in **Fig. 3**).

When considering the various reconstruction techniques available in the literature, although the fibular sling technique has shown positive outcomes, this approach attempts to recreate function of the FCL and PFL while failing to address the PLT.[42] This is why the authors recommend using an anatomic-based reconstruction technique for restoring all 3 major structures of the PLC (PFL, PLT, and FCL) to restore normal knee function and kinematics.

DEVELOPMENT OF AN ANATOMIC-BASED RECONSTRUCTION TECHNIQUES
Reinforcement by Research

To further improve treatment of PLC injuries requiring surgical management, LaPrade and colleagues[43] used quantitative anatomic[1] and biomechanical[25,44] studies for development of a PLC reconstruction technique that would best replicate the native features of these structures Previously, the anatomic characteristics of the PLC relative to the native attachment sites and orientation of the structures that formed the

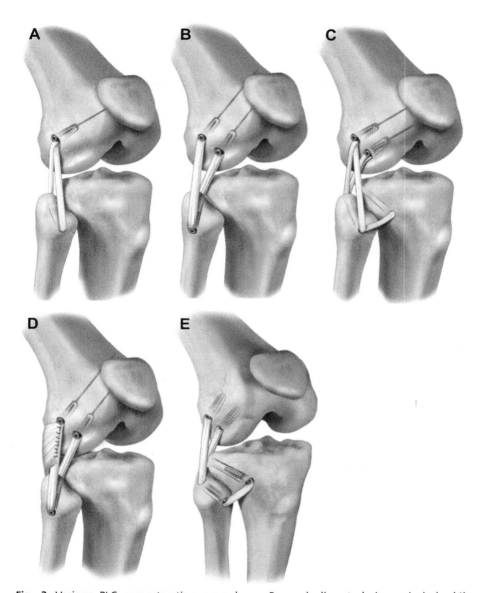

Fig. 3. Various PLC reconstruction procedures. Femoral sling techniques include (*A*) 1-femoral tunnel fibular sling technique and (*B*) 2-femoral tunnel fibular sling technique. PLC reconstruction with 2 grafts (*C*) with 1 graft recreating the FCL with a fibular sling and the second graft recreating the PLT and PFL with a graft strand overlying the anterior tibiofibular joint. Posterolateral capsular shift with a fibular sling (*D*), attaching the postero-lateral capsule to the FCL graft (*E*). PLC reconstruction with 1 graft recreating the FCL, PLT, and PFL. (*From* Moulton SG, Geeslin AG, LaPrade RF, et al. A systematic review of the out-comes of posterolateral corner knee injuries, part 2: surgical treatment of chronic injuries. Am J Sports Med 2016;44:1616–23; with permission.)

basis of this anatomic reconstruction technique were discussed. A biomechanical study was then performed to determine the tensile strength of each main static stabilizing PLC structure, to narrow the selection for the most optimal graft choice for both a complete PLC reconstruction and for isolated FCL and PLT reconstructions.[44–47]

After restoration of the native structural features and anatomic attachment sites of the PLC, the authors' technique was then tested for validation of static knee stabilization. The anatomic-based reconstruction of the FCL, PFL, and PLT developed was found to restore both static varus and external rotation stability and also not result in over-constraint of the knee[27] (which was a common problem with the non–anatomic-based reconstructions at the time). Additionally, relative to an earlier study determining human ligament graft strengths,[44,45] LaPrade and colleagues determined that an autogenous semitendinosus graft was most the ideal graft choice due to sufficient strength in replication of FCL tensile strength and increased length, while additionally reducing the chance of saphenous nerve irritation during harvest.

A follow-up multicenter prospective outcomes study[26] further validated this procedure by finding that anatomic PLC reconstruction yielded improved both subjective and objective patient outcomes as well as improved knee stability at an average follow-up of 4.3 years.

Isolated Posterolateral Corner Reconstructions

Further studies then performed anatomic-based analyses of both isolated FCL and PLT reconstructions. Coobs and colleagues[25] used a semitendinosus graft that coursed between tunnels positioned at the anatomic attachment sites of the FCL on the femur and fibular head (**Fig. 4**). The graft passed medial to both the superficial layer of the iliotibial band and the lateral aponeurosis of the long head of the biceps femoris.[12] The graft was then fixed at 30° of knee flexion, which was chosen because the greatest amount of varus instability is seen at this degree of knee flexion in biomechanical models[2,3] in addition to the greatest forces seen in ACL grafts on FCL sectioning.[10] In this biomechanical model, the deviation in varus, external, and internal rotation that occurs on isolated FCL injuries was successfully restored to near normal knee stability.

A subsequent biomechanical study was conducted for analyzing the reconstruction of the PLT after simulated sectioning/injury. This biomechanical study recreated the PLT by using the surgical approach described by Terry and LaPrade.[12] This reconstruction technique anatomically reconstructs the PLT by identifying its femoral attachment at the proximal portion of the anterior fifth of the popliteal sulcus of the femur while avoiding the nearby FCL attachment located just posterior and proximal (**Fig. 5**).[1] A 7-mm diameter tunnel is then reamed to a depth of 25 mm over a guide pin that was previously drilled across to the anteromedial knee, which exited just proximal and anterior to the adductor tubercle. A transtibial tunnel was then created by locating the flat area just distal and medial to Gerdy tubercle and guiding a 7-mm reamer through to the musculotendinous junction on the posterior tibia. At various knee flexion angles, this procedure significantly reduced the increase in external rotation that occurs after PLT sectioning; however, full restoration of internal rotation, varus angulation, and anterior translation was unable to be obtained.

Anatomic Posterolateral Corner Reconstruction Technique

An anatomic reconstruction procedure was detailed by LaPrade and colleagues,[27] in which they identify the attachment sites and reproduction of PLC static function while using a split Achilles tendon allograft (**Fig. 6**). The tibial and fibular tunnels are drilled at the midpoint of their attachment sites (detailed previously). The attachment site of the

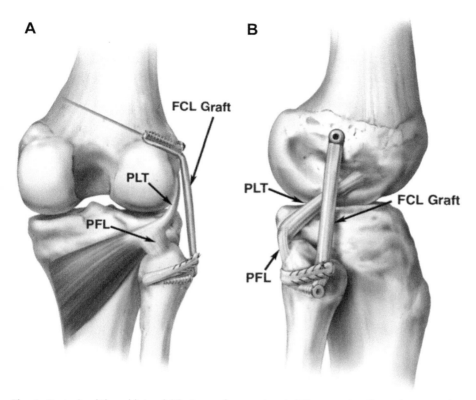

A

B

Fig. 4. Posterior (*A*) and lateral (*B*) views of an anatomic FCL reconstruction using a semitendinosous graft on a right knee. The fibular tunnel is recreated distal to the fibular attachment of the PFL, whereas the femoral tunnel is recreated slightly proximal and posterior to the lateral epicondyle. (*From* Coobs BR, LaPrade RF, Griffith CJ, et al. Biomechanical analysis of an isolated fibular (lateral) collateral ligament reconstruction using an autogenous semitendinosus graft. Am J Sports Med 2007;35:1523; with permission.)

FCL on the lateral aspect of the fibular head is drilled through by a guide pin, followed by a 7-mm reamer to the attachment site of the PFL on the posteromedial fibular styloid. The transtibial tunnel for the PLT is then created in the same fashion as the isolated reconstruction procedure detailed by LaPrade and collagues[8] (described previously). This is followed with two 9-mm parallel femoral tunnels at the FCL and PLT attachment sites, directed anteromedially and exiting proximomedially to the medial epicondyle and adductor tubercle (avoiding the ACL and PCL graft tunnels in case of multiligament procedures).

The bone plug of the first graft is first secured at the proximal half and anterior fifth of the popliteus sulcus, recreating the PLT, and is then passed distally along the popliteal hiatus and pulled through the tibial tunnel at the posterolateral aspect of the lateral tibial plateau. The second graft is used to reconstruct both the FCL and PFL, beginning with an initial fixation at the femoral attachment of the FCL, followed by passing of the graft medial (deep to) to the superficial layer of the iliotibial band and anterior arm of the long head of the biceps femoris to the tunnel of the fibular head where the graft is passed posterior to anterior. After the FCL is

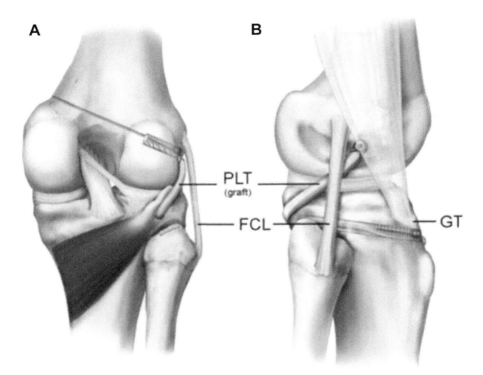

Fig. 5. Posterior (*A*) and lateral (*B*) views of an isolated anatomic PLT reconstruction using a semitendinosus graft on a right knee. The proximal portion of the of the anterior fifth of the popliteal sulcus is the site for the femoral attachment. The tibial attachment is recreated from reaming a tunnel located at a flat area just distal and medial to Gerdy tubercle (GT) and exiting on the posterior tibia near the musculotendinous junction. (*From* LaPrade RF, Wozniczka JK, Stellmaker MP, et al. Analysis of the static function of the popliteus tendon and evaluation of an anatomic reconstruction: the "fifth ligament" of the knee. Am J Sports Med 2010;38:545; with permission.)

recreated from fixation at the fibular tunnel, the remaining portion of the graft is passed proximomedially to the posterolateral tibial tunnel located at the popliteus musculotendinous junction and pulled through posterior to anterior. Both grafts through this tunnel are then tightened and fixed with the knee in 60° of knee flexion and 5° of internal rotation.

SUMMARY

Isolated or combined treatments for the PLC of the knee are most optimally treated in the acute stage (<3 weeks) after injury, while individual anatomic structures are still identifiable. If surgical management is necessary (grade III injuries), and the injuries are able to be managed in the acute setting, repair of avulsion injuries has been shown to yield positive patient outcomes, in addition to low failure rates. Once the injury has transitioned to a more chronic state (>3 weeks), however, reconstruction is the preferred treatment method. More specifically, anatomic reconstruction of the FCL, PLT, and PFL based on their native anatomic attachment sites is the

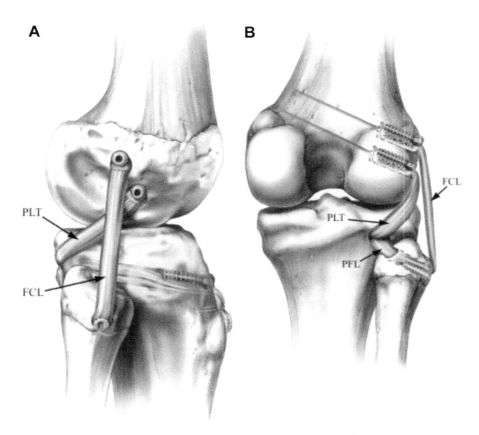

Fig. 6. Illustration of the anatomic PLC reconstruction in the (*A*) lateral and (*B*) posterior views of a right knee. This reconstruction incorporates 2 grafts for recreating the 3 major structures of the PLC. (*From* LaPradeRF, Johansen S, Wentorf FA, et al. An analysis of an anatomical posterolateral knee reconstruction: an in vitro biomechanical study and development of a surgical technique. Am J Sports Med 2004;32:1410; with permission.)

most optimal treatment to provide patients with a stable knee and a successful outcome.

REFERENCES

1. LaPrade RF, Ly TV, Wentorf FA, et al. The posterolateral attachments of the knee: a qualitative and quantitative morphologic analysis of the fibular collateral ligament, popliteus tendon, popliteofibular ligament, and lateral gastrocnemius tendon. Am J Sports Med 2003;31:854–60.

2. Gollehon DL, Torzilli PA, Warren RF. The role of the posterolateral and cruciate ligaments in the stability of the human knee. A biomechanical study. J Bone Joint Surg Am 1987;69:233–42.

3. Grood ES, Stowers SF, Noyes FR. Limits of movement in the human knee. Effect of sectioning the posterior cruciate ligament and posterolateral structures. J Bone Joint Surg Am 1988;70:88–97.

4. LaPrade RF, Tso A, Wentorf FA. Force measurements on the fibular collateral ligament, popliteofibular ligament, and popliteus tendon to applied loads. Am J Sports Med 2004;32:1695–701.

5. Gwathmey FW Jr, Tompkins MA, Gaskin CM, et al. Can stress radiography of the knee help characterize posterolateral corner injury. Clin Orthop Relat Res 2012; 470:768–73.

6. Ranawat A, Baker CL 3rd, Henry S, et al. Posterolateral corner injury of the knee: evaluation and management. J Am Acad Orthop Surg 2008;16:506–18.

7. Parsons EM, Gee AO, Spiekerman C, et al. The biomechanical function of the anterolateral ligament of the knee: response. Am J Sports Med 2015;43:NP22.

8. LaPrade RF, Wozniczka JK, Stellmaker MP, et al. Analysis of the static function of the popliteus tendon and evaluation of an anatomic reconstruction: the "fifth ligament" of the knee. Am J Sports Med 2010;38:543–9.

9. LaPrade RF. Arthroscopic evaluation of the lateral compartment of knees with grade 3 posterolateral knee complex injuries. Am J Sports Med 1997;25: 596–602.

10. LaPrade RF, Resig S, Wentorf F, et al. The effects of grade III posterolateral knee complex injuries on anterior cruciate ligament graft force. A biomechanical analysis. Am J Sports Med 1999;27:469–75.

11. Geeslin AG, LaPrade RF. Location of bone bruises and other osseous injuries associated with acute grade III isolated and combined posterolateral knee injuries. Am J Sports Med 2010;38:2502–8.

12. Terry GC, LaPrade RF. The posterolateral aspect of the knee. Anatomy and surgical approach. Am J Sports Med 1996;24:732–9.

13. Moatshe G, Dornan G, Loken S, et al. Demographics and injuries associated with knee dislocation: a prospective review of 303 patients. Orthop J Sports Med 2017;5. 2325967117706521.

14. Kannus P. Nonoperative treatment of grade II and III sprains of the lateral ligament compartment of the knee. Am J Sports Med 1989;17:83–8.

15. DeLee JC, Riley MB, Rockwood CA Jr. Acute straight lateral instability of the knee. Am J Sports Med 1983;11:404–11.

16. Grana WA, Janssen T. Lateral ligament injury of the knee. Orthopedics 1987;10: 1039–44.

17. Krukhaug Y, Molster A, Rodt A, et al. Lateral ligament injuries of the knee. Knee Surg Sports Traumatol Arthrosc 1998;6:21–5.

18. Stannard JP, Brown SL, Farris RC, et al. The posterolateral corner of the knee: repair versus reconstruction. Am J Sports Med 2005;33:881–8.

19. Pietrini SD, LaPrade RF, Griffith CJ, et al. Radiographic identification of the primary posterolateral knee structures. Am J Sports Med 2009;37:542–51.

20. Levy BA, Dajani KA, Morgan JA, et al. Repair versus reconstruction of the fibular collateral ligament and posterolateral corner in the multiligament-injured knee. Am J Sports Med 2010;38:804–9.

21. Geeslin AG, LaPrade RF. Outcomes of treatment of acute grade-III isolated and combined posterolateral knee injuries: a prospective case series and surgical technique. J Bone Joint Surg Am 2011;93:1672–83.

22. Baker CL Jr, Norwood LA, Hughston JC. Acute posterolateral rotatory instability of the knee. J Bone Joint Surg Am 1983;65:614–8.

23. DeLee JC, Riley MB, Rockwood CA Jr. Acute posterolateral rotatory instability of the knee. Am J Sports Med 1983;11:199–207.

24. LaPrade RF, Hamilton CD, L. E. Treatment or acute and chronic combined anterior cruciate ligament and posterolateral knee ligament injuries. Sports Med Arthrosc 1997;5:91–9.

25. Coobs BR, LaPrade RF, Griffith CJ, et al. Biomechanical analysis of an isolated fibular (lateral) collateral ligament reconstruction using an autogenous semitendinosus graft. Am J Sports Med 2007;35:1521–7.

26. LaPrade RF, Johansen S, Agel J, et al. Outcomes of an anatomic posterolateral knee reconstruction. J Bone Joint Surg Am 2010;92:16–22.

27. LaPrade RF, Johansen S, Wentorf FA, et al. An analysis of an anatomical posterolateral knee reconstruction: an in vitro biomechanical study and development of a surgical technique. Am J Sports Med 2004;32:1405–14.

28. Baker CL Jr, Norwood LA, Hughston JC. Acute combined posterior cruciate and posterolateral instability of the knee. Am J Sports Med 1984;12:204–8.

29. Neuschwander DC, Drez D Jr, Paine RM. Simultaneous high tibial osteotomy and ACL reconstruction for combined genu varum and symptomatic ACL tear. Orthopedics 1993;16:679–84.

30. Noyes FR, Barber-Westin SD, Hewett TE. High tibial osteotomy and ligament reconstruction for varus angulated anterior cruciate ligament-deficient knees. Am J Sports Med 2000;28:282–96.

31. Arthur A, LaPrade RF, Agel J. Proximal tibial opening wedge osteotomy as the initial treatment for chronic posterolateral corner deficiency in the varus knee: a prospective clinical study. Am J Sports Med 2007;35:1844–50.

32. Geeslin AG, Moulton SG, LaPrade RF. A systematic review of the outcomes of posterolateral corner knee injuries, part 1: surgical treatment of acute injuries. Am J Sports Med 2016;44:1336–42.

33. Fanelli GC, Fanelli DG, Edson CJ, et al. Combined anterior cruciate ligament and posterolateral reconstruction of the knee using allograft tissue in chronic knee injuries. J Knee Surg 2014;27:353–8.

34. Jakobsen BW, Lund B, Christiansen SE, et al. Anatomic reconstruction of the posterolateral corner of the knee: a case series with isolated reconstructions in 27 patients. Arthroscopy 2010;26:918–25.

35. Schechinger SJ, Levy BA, Dajani KA, et al. Achilles tendon allograft reconstruction of the fibular collateral ligament and posterolateral corner. Arthroscopy 2009; 25:232–42.

36. Yoon KH, Lee JH, Bae DK, et al. Comparison of clinical results of anatomic posterolateral corner reconstruction for posterolateral rotatory instability of the knee with or without popliteal tendon reconstruction. Am J Sports Med 2011; 39:2421–8.

37. Zorzi C, Alam M, Iacono V, et al. Combined PCL and PLC reconstruction in chronic posterolateral instability. Knee Surg Sports Traumatol Arthrosc 2013;21: 1036–42.

38. Kim SJ, Choi DH, Hwang BY. The influence of posterolateral rotatory instability on ACL reconstruction: comparison between isolated ACL reconstruction and ACL reconstruction combined with posterolateral corner reconstruction. J Bone Joint Surg Am 2012;94:253–9.

39. Kim SJ, Jung M, Moon HK, et al. Anterolateral transtibial posterior cruciate ligament reconstruction combined with anatomical reconstruction of posterolateral corner insufficiency: comparison of single-bundle versus double-bundle posterior cruciate ligament reconstruction over a 2- to 6-year follow-up. Am J Sports Med 2011;39:481–9.

40. Kim SJ, Kim SG, Lee IS, et al. Effect of physiological posterolateral rotatory laxity on early results of posterior cruciate ligament reconstruction with posterolateral corner reconstruction. J Bone Joint Surg Am 2013;95:1222–7.
41. Kim SJ, Chang JH, Kang YH, et al. Clinical comparison of anteromedial versus anterolateral tibial tunnel direction for transtibial posterior cruciate ligament reconstruction: 2 to 8 years' follow-up. Am J Sports Med 2009;37:693–8.
42. Arciero RA. Anatomic posterolateral corner knee reconstruction. Arthroscopy 2005;21:1147.
43. LaPrade RF, Griffith CJ, Coobs BR, et al. Improving outcomes for posterolateral knee injuries. J Orthop Res 2014;32:485–91.
44. LaPrade RF, Bollom TS, Wentorf FA, et al. Mechanical properties of the posterolateral structures of the knee. Am J Sports Med 2005;33:1386–91.
45. Noyes FR, Butler DL, Grood ES, et al. Biomechanical analysis of human ligament grafts used in knee-ligament repairs and reconstructions. J Bone Joint Surg Am 1984;66:344–52.
46. Hunter LY, Louis DS, Ricciardi JR, et al. The saphenous nerve: its course and importance in medial arthrotomy. Am J Sports Med 1979;7:227–30.
47. Worth RM, Kettelkamp DB, Defalque RJ, et al. Saphenous nerve entrapment. A cause of medial knee pain. Am J Sports Med 1984;12:80–1.

Repair and Augmentation with Internal Brace in the Multiligament Injured Knee

John Dabis, MBBS, MRCS, FRCS (Tr&Orth), MSc, SEM[a],*,
Adrian Wilson, MBBS, MRCS, FRCS (Tr&Orth)[b,1,2]

KEYWORDS

- Ligament augmentation • Internal brace • Ligament reinforcement
- Multiligament knee injury • Ligament repair

KEY POINTS

- Multiligament knee injuries are part of a complex spectrum of knee injuries. It is important to clinically assess the common peroneal nerve, vasculature of the limb, and integrity of the ligamentous structures.
- Internal brace ligament augmentation is a concept that can assist ligament repair. It is a bridging concept using braided suture tape and knotless bone anchors to reinforce ligament strength, acting as a secondary stabilizer after repair.
- Early evidence suggests improved clinical outcomes with ligament reconstruction; however, with improved suture material and implants, ligament suture repair can provide equally successful outcomes.
- Anterior cruciate ligament repair has shown some promising early results, especially in the pediatric group, with low rerupture rates, high level of return to preinjury level of activity, and no growth disturbance.
- Techniques of internal bracing, such as primary medial collateral ligament repair, are minimally invasive, preserve native anatomy, are technically straightforward, and allow immediate rehabilitation because the repair is protected by the internal brace.

Disclosures: All named authors hereby declare that they have no conflicts of interest to disclose and we did not receive funding for this research.
[a] Department of Orthopaedics, Brisbane Private Hospital, Level 6, Specialist Centre, 259 Wickham Terrace, Spring Hill, QLD 4000, Australia; [b] The Wellington and Portland Children's Hospitals, Queen Anne Street Medical Centre, 18-22, Queen Anne Street, London W1G 8HU, UK
[1] Present address: 18-22 Queen Anne Street, London W1G 8HU, UK.
[2] Senior author.
* Corresponding author. 42 Golf Side, South Cheam, Surrey, London SM2 7EZ, UK.
E-mail address: johndabis1@gmail.com

DIAGNOSIS

Multiligament knee injuries (MLKIs) can be caused by both high-energy trauma, such as road traffic accidents and falls from height, and low-energy trauma, including sporting activities.[1] The nomenclature needs to be well-defined. Knee dislocations often result in MLKIs but not all MLKIs are dislocations. Patterns of injury are clear from the history; varus and valgus loads with or without contact are a common presenting complaint. Sudden torsion or hyperextension can be part of the injury spectrum. The clinician should have a high level of suspicion for the MLKI based on the mechanism of injury. For high-energy injuries Advanced trauma life support principles apply and are the initial priority. Vigilance is required because MLKIs often lead to a dislocation and this can spontaneously reduce postinjury or on transfer. A thorough clinical neurologic examination should be performed to exclude a common peroneal nerve palsy. Up to one-third of posterolateral corner (PLC) injuries sustain a concomitant common peroneal nerve injury.[2,3] Because more than 70% of PLC injuries occur with associated cruciate ligament injuries, all aspects of the ligamentous, neurologic, and vascular integrity need to be interrogated. Foot pulses and skin color should be monitored and documented. Vascular assessment is critical because the risk of popliteal artery injury can be as high as 44%.[4] Normal and symmetric pulses and capillary refill can provide valuable information. The specificity and sensitivity of ankle-brachial index (ABPI) assessment in MLKI are well documented.[5] The systolic arterial pressure of the injured limb is divided by the systolic arterial pressure of the uninjured limb; ABPI less than 0.9 is indicative of arterial injury.

Further detailed information with MRI should be ascertained. Valuable information can be sourced from stress radiographs. Varus stress radiographs demonstrating greater than 2.7 mm to 4 mm side-to-side difference between the injured and noninjured sides indicate an isolated fibular collateral ligament tear whereas greater than 4 mm indicates a complete PLC injury. Valgus stress radiographs demonstrating a side-to-side difference of 3.2 mm to 9.8 mm demonstrate complete disruption to the superficial medial collateral ligament (sMCL). Greater than 9.8 mm difference demonstrates complete disruption to all the medial structures. Kneeling stress radiographs also can provide useful information about the integrity of the posterior cruciate ligament (PCL). A posterior translational side-to-side difference of up to 6 mm demonstrates a partial injury, whereas an 8 mm to 11 mm difference indicates an isolated complete PCL tear and greater than 12 mm difference implies a PCL rupture as part of an MLKI, such as an associated PLC or posteromedial corner (PMC) injury.[6,7]

CONCEPTS OF INTERNAL BRACE

The concept of internal brace ligament augmentation (IBLA) was popularized by Mackay and colleagues.[8] The concept is based on a ligament repair bridging concept using braided ultra–high-molecular-weight polyethylene/polyester suture tape to allow mobilization during early-phase healing. It is believed to act as a secondary stabilizer and work as a check rein that is only loaded at the end of range.

CLINICAL MANAGEMENT

van Eck and colleagues[9] performed a systematic review of the literature to assess if there is a role for internal bracing and repair of the anterior cruciate ligament (ACL). Clinical studies were reviewed and factors that could influence the outcome, such as tear type and location, fixation technique, and suture material were evaluated. The primary outcomes of interest for the clinical studies were the revision rate, anterior laxity, and pivot shift. Secondary outcome measures included patient-reported outcome measures (PROMs) and patient satisfaction. More recent preclinical studies on ACL repair have shown the strength of the repair improved when nonabsorbable sutures were used. Fisher and colleagues[10] tested the biomechanical properties of internal bracing of the ACL repair in a goat model. Anterior tibial translation was closer to the intact state when internal bracing was added to the ACL repair. Wilson and colleagues,[11] Smith and colleagues,[12] and Eggli and colleagues[13] all published small case series of ACL internal bracing.

Internal bracing is a concept and technique used in ligament repair. Several concepts have evolved, however, from using ultra–high-molecular-weight polyethylene/polyester suture tape within ligament repair and reconstruction. Several surgical techniques[14–17] have been published mainly describing the technique of internal suture augmentation. Graft reinforcement is a novel distinct entity, which the senior author has been using since 2011. It is a concept and technique of using a high-strain suture tape, FiberTape (Arthrex, Naples, Florida), to reinforce ligament reconstructions around the knee. Short-term functional PROMs and results of a series of 282 patients are in the process of publication. Indications for intra-articular reinforcement include the following:

- All PCL reconstructions
- All allografts
- All grafts of less than 8 mm in diameter
- All revisions
- All hypermobile patients
- Use in elite athletes

Extra-articular reconstruction indications include PLC reconstructions and some medial patellofemoral ligament (MPFL) reconstructions.

Anterior Cruciate Ligament Repair and Augmentation

Aboalata and colleagues[16] elegantly present internal suture augmentation to protect the all-inside ACL reconstruction surgical technique.[18,19] The ultra–high-molecular-weight polyethylene/polyester tape is fixed on both the femoral and tibial buttons in an all-inside manner. A backup fixation with a BioKnotless (Arthrex, Naples, Florida) anchor is added distal to the exit of the tibial socket. Two adjustable cortical suspensory devices are used on both the femoral and tibial sides. A single semitendinosus tendon harvest is performed and quadrupled for the preparation of a GraftLink (Arthrex, Naples, Florida) construct. A quadrupled semitendinosus graft rarely yields a graft diameter of less than 8 mm. This single-bundle anatomic ACL reconstruction is performed by using a FlipCutter (Arthrex, Naples, Florida) to create the retrosockets in a retrograde fashion after introduction through an outside-in maneuver. The graft is passed into the femoral socket initially by pulling of the traction sutures, followed by graft advancement and docking by synching down the white sutures (TightRope, Arthrex). The fixation is backed up by passing the internal suture augmentation tape tails (FiberTape) in a bioabsorbable bone anchor (SwiveLock, Arthrex), which is subsequently anchored into the anteromedial tibia distal to the tibial tunnel.

This method of internal brace suture augmentation to protect the ACL reconstruction graft also can be performed using a cortical suspensory button device on the femur and a Bio-Interference (Arthrex, Naples, Florida) screw on the tibial side.[17] The tibial tunnel can be completed and all the sutures, including the internal suture augmentation tails, are tensioned under 80 N of traction with the knee in 30° of flexion, valgus position, and the foot in external rotation. Several options are available for the internal suture augmentation tails, including a bone anchor, cortical button, staple, or 6.5 mm cancellous screw.

MacKay and colleagues[8] reviewed the PROMs and reoperation rates of a technique of ACL repair that combined repair with a synthetic IBLA; 68 of the 82 cohort patients were suitable to undergo a repair with the IBLA; however, only 27 patients had a complete data set of PROMs (1-year follow-up). Surgery was performed within 3 months of the original injury. The ACL remnant was whipstitched using an arthroscopic suture passing instrument. The proximal end of the ACL was then reapproximated against the medial wall of the lateral femoral condyle, in an anatomic midbundle position. Discussion of the position of ideal femoral footprint is outside the scope of this article. The side wall of the condyle is freshened with a microfracture probe. The internal brace is then passed through 3.5 mm tunnels in the femur and tibia. Proximal femoral fixation was secured with a TightRope while distal tibial fixation of the internal brace was carried out with the SwiveLock suture anchor. The cumulative reintervention rate for rerupture was 1.5%. The PROMs, including the Knee Injury and Osteoarthritis Outcome Score and Western Ontario and McMaster Universities Osteoarthritis Index, all had statistical significant improvement after 3 months and continued to be the case 1-year postoperatively.

Smith and colleagues[12] have reported on 3 pediatric ACL direct repairs using the internal brace method. A modification to the surgical technique described by MacKay and colleagues[8] was used for 2 additional cases. An all-epiphyseal technique with 2.4 mm diameter intra-epiphyseal femoral and tibial tunnels was used. A looped shuttling suture was passed into the joint through each tunnel and retrieved through the anteromedial (AM) portal. The loop of the femoral suture was divided resulting in 2 snare sutures: 1 suture was used to deliver the ACL repair sutures back through the femoral tunnel; the other snare was attached to the tibial looped suture, which was introduced through the native ACL and pulled through the tibial tunnel. This shuttling suture was then used to advance the internal brace. Further short-term 2-year PROMs and results of 22 pediatric ACL repairs with a modified surgical technique are in the process of publication.

Medial Collateral Ligament Repair and Augmentation

Medial-sided knee injuries are common; however, a majority of medial-sided knee injuries do not require surgical treatment. Grade III injuries or combined MLKIs may require surgical stabilization. Gilmer and colleagues[20] performed a biomechanical analysis using 27 matched cadaveric knees, 9 pairs per assay. Assay 1 compared anatomic repair with internal bracing with the intact state. Assay 2 compared repair alone with internal bracing, and assay 3 compared anatomic repair with internal bracing with allograft reconstruction. Valgus load was applied and failure was the endpoint. Stiffness and valgus displacement angles were measured.

The medial side of the knee was dissected, and particular care was taken to identify the entire medial collateral ligament (MCL) and posterior oblique ligament (POL), medial epicondyle and adductor tubercle, and tibial insertion of the semimembranosus. Repair was performed using 2 suture anchors loaded with high-strength suture at the anatomic MCL and POL femoral footprints. Internal bracing was performed by loading a high-strength suture tie (FiberTape; Arthrex) into each of the anchors at the femoral MCL and POL footprints. The suture tie from the MCL anchor was secured to the anatomic tibial insertion of the MCL. The suture tie from the POL anchor was secured to the anatomic tibial footprint of the POL. Care was taken not to over-constrain the repair. Reconstruction was performed using 2 bovine tendon allografts, as described by LaPrade.[21] The results demonstrated for assay 1 were as follows: the mean moment for internal bracing was significantly less than the intact state; however, the mean valgus angle at failure was not significantly different than for the intact state. The results demonstrated for assay 2 were as follows: the mean moment for internal bracing was significantly greater than for repair, and the mean valgus angle at failure was significantly greater than for repair. The results demonstrated for assay 3 were as follows: the mean moment for internal bracing was not significantly different than for reconstruction neither was there a difference in the the mean valgus angle at failure; when comparing internal bracing with repair alone, the moment to failure was significantly greater for internal bracing, and valgus angle at failure was significantly less, suggesting the ability of the knee to resist deformity.

Anatomy of the MCL is crucial in reconstruction. The sMCL has 1 femoral and 2 tibial attachments. The femoral attachment of the sMCL is slightly oval in shape and is located in a depression that was an average 3.2 mm proximal and 4.8 mm posterior to the medial epicondyle. As the sMCL courses distally, it has 2 separate tibial attachments. The proximal attachment of the sMCL is primarily to soft tissues rather than directly to bone. The majority of the soft tissue deep to the proximal tibial attachment of the sMCL was the anterior arm of the semimembranosus tendon, which itself is attached to bone. The distal tibial attachment is broad based and is located anterior to the posteromedial crest of the tibia.

The POL consists of 3 fascial attachments that course off the distal aspect of the semimembranosus tendon at the knee: superficial, central, and capsular arms. The POL attaches on average 7.7 mm distal and 6.4 mm posterior to the adductor tubercle and 1.4 mm distal and 2.9 mm anterior to the gastrocnemius tubercle. The central arm is the thickest and largest portion of the POL. It courses from the distal aspect of the semimembranosus tendon and has thick fascial reinforcement of both meniscofemoral and meniscotibial portions of the posteromedial capsule. The distal tibial attachment site of the sMCL is deep within the pes anserine bursa, 6 cm distal to the joint line. The POL tibial site of attachment is to replicate the central arm of the POL and is identified slightly anterior to the direct arm attachment of the semimembranosus tendon.

Lubowitz and colleagues[22] described a MCL and PMC anatomic repair with internal bracing. Deep dissection to identify the anatomic landmarks is critical. If there is any doubt as to the positions of the critical landmarks, an isometry test can be performed. A 1.6 mm guide pin is inserted into the MCL femoral origin proximal and posterior to the medial femoral epicondyle. The tibial guide pin is inserted only after identifying the MCL and POL insertions, and the tibial insertion of the semimembranosus tendon. The exact insertion point should be within the posterior fibers of the tibial sMCL, which is located 6-cm distal to the joint line. To construct the internal brace, a high-strength suture is loaded on the femoral anchor before anchor insertion. After the femoral-sided repair is complete, internal brace augmentation is performed by tensioning the suture tape while inserting the tibial suture anchor at the MCL tibial footprint.

van der List and colleagues[23] described their surgical technique of a minimally invasive MCL internal brace. An MRI is suggested preoperatively to identify which medial structures are ruptured. The first stage is to perform a primary MCL repair. A 4 cm longitudinal incision is made over the medial epicondyle and carried down through layer 1. The most common site of injury is the femoral side. The proximal and retracted avulsed MCL should be identified. An interlocking Bunnell-pattern suturing is performed. The femoral origin of the sMCL is then identified and a bone anchor (4.75 mm vented BioComposite SwiveLock suture anchor [Arthrex]) is inserted proximal and posterior to the medial epicondyle with the repair sutures through the eyelet. The ultra–high-molecular-weight polyethyelene/polyester suture tape (FiberTape) is also inserted through the eyelet before being deployed. The second stage is to complete the internal brace for the sMCL. For this, a second incision over the tibial insertion, which is located 6-cm distal to the joint line, is made. Dissection to identify the distal fibers of the MCL is made. A curved artery clamp to tunneled deep to layer one, creating a subcutaneous tunnel, to exit the proximal wound. The suture tape is then channeled under the skin bridge along the repaired sMCL and should be anchored down at the distal insertion site of the sMCL. The most important factors, at this stage, are the position of the knee at tensioning and to not over-constrain or under-constrain the knee. The suture tape should be tensioned with the knee in 30° of flexion. The bone anchor can be partially deployed and the knee examined for range of movement and valgus instability. Final adjustments then can be made. Neutral rotation of the tibia is ideal. The knee should be kept in varus to prevent gapping of the joint medially. To avoid over-constraint, a small instrument, such as a hemostat, can be placed under the suture tie during anchor implantation.

Kovachevich and colleagues[24] performed a systematic review of the literature for the outcomes of surgical management of the MCL in the setting of an MLKI. After selection of specific inclusion criteria (English, human subjects, and mean follow-up of 24 months), 8 articles were identified that were all level IV evidence. Five articles reported on MCL repair and 3 on MCL reconstruction. There were no articles comparing MCL repair with reconstruction at this time. Of the limited evidence, repair and reconstruction both yield satisfactory results. More recently,[25] a small cohort study presented the medium-term patient reported outcomes after MLKIs comparing MCL repair with reconstruction. Patients undergoing MCL repair generally had higher PROMs than those undergoing reconstructions at a mean 6-year follow-up. The repair technique was performed using anchors and sutures. The PMC and POL were then mobilized and imbricated anteriorly using a pants-over-vest technique. Reconstruction used nonirradiated semitendinosus allografts. They did not compare the use of the internal brace with reconstruction.

Posterior Cruciate Ligament and Posterolateral Corner Repair and Augmentation

PLC injury management has evolved over the past 2 decades. Repair was the gold standard until Stannard and colleagues[26] demonstrated significantly higher failure rates in patients who underwent repair compared with reconstruction. Levy and colleagues[27] validated this, showing similar findings. There has been a recent resurgence of early intervention compared with delayed reconstruction,[28] and this is echoed throughout the literature.[29] Surgical reconstruction is recommended for grade III PLC injuries.[30] In a recent systematic review,[31] several surgical techniques were described, including the anatomic-based PLC reconstruction and the fibular sling technique; however, there are no case series that described an internal brace repair technique. Geeslin and colleagues,[31] in this systematic review, did establish that repair of grade III PLC injuries and staged treatment of combined cruciate injuries were associated with a substantially higher postoperative PLC failure rate.

MacKay and colleagues[8] have presented their experience with PCL and PLC internal brace with no adverse effects. The senior author's surgical preference for PCL reconstruction is a single-bundle reinforced peroneus longus allograft GraftLink PCL reconstruction with back-up fixation on the ultra–high-molecular-weight suture tape. The senior author has published 2 arthroscopic techniques on PCL reconstruction.[32,33]

Trasolini and Rick Hatch[34] described an all-arthroscopic technique for suture augmentation of incomplete PCL injuries that preserve the native anatomy and ligament balance while allowing for accelerated rehabilitation. A 70° arthroscope from the posteromedial portal is used to evaluate the PCL. If incomplete tears were seen, with a significant percentage of fibers intact, internal bracing would be performed. The interval adjacent to the medial femoral condyle in the intercondylar notch is used. The posterior septum is divided and the space posterior to the PCL tibial insertion site is developed. The tibial tunnel is created with the aid of fluoroscopic assistance. The femoral tunnel is created and an anterolateral-bundle position is adopted, which is juxta-articular. The instruments used for the preparation of the suture augmentation device is a combination of the FiberTape and TightRope (Arthrex). The RetroButton (Arthrex, Naples, Florida) is passed through the intact PCL ligament and into the femoral tunnel. The internal brace is then pulled through via a TigerStick (Arthrex, Naples, Florida) and tensioned with a 4.75 mm BioComposite SwiveLock. Tension is maintained in 90° of flexion ensuring over-reduction is not performed.

Frosch and colleagues[35,36] performed a meta-analysis comparing suture repair of the cruciates versus reconstruction in the setting of knee dislocations. The difficulty arises due to the lack of homogeneity in the injury pattern after knee dislocations. Levy and colleagues'[37] systematic review demonstrated decreased stability, reduced range of movement, and a lower return to preinjury activity level in the cruciate repair group compared with the reconstruction group. Autologous tendon reconstruction of the cruciate ligaments yielded superior results compared with those undergoing suture repair. Frosch and colleagues[35] accounted for injury pattern with respect to the Schenck[38] classification and compared the clinical outcome of ACL and PCL suture repair with nonoperative treatment. Suture repair outcomes were significantly better because 70% of the nonoperative patient cohort resulted in moderate or poor outcomes. Likewise, the reconstruction group showed improved outcomes compared with the nonoperative group. No significant difference was found in clinical outcome when comparing the ligament suture and reconstruction groups; 77.5% of patients with Schenck III and IV knee dislocations undergoing suture repair demonstrated good and excellent clinical outcomes.

Internal bracing does not come without risk. Concerns continue about the risk of over-constraint of the knee with internal bracing, which may lead to premature osteoarthritis; hence, care must be taken when tensioning the construct.

SUMMARY

Internal bracing is a technique that all surgeons treating MLKIs should be aware of. It provides a robust stable repair to the knee joint and allows the tissues to bridge while promoting early rehabilitation. This inevitably avoids joint stiffness due to restricted or protected range of joint movement.

REFERENCES

1. Engebretsen L, Risberg MA, Robertson B, et al. Outcome after knee dislocations: a 2-9 years follow-up of 85 consecutive patients. Knee Surg Sports Traumatol Arthrosc 2009;17(9):1013–26.
2. Moatshe G, Dornan GJ, Løken S, et al. Demographics and injuries associated with knee dislocation: a prospective review of 303 patients. Orthop J Sports Med 2017;5(5). 2325967117706521.
3. Niall DM, Nutton RW, Keating JF. Palsy of the common peroneal nerve after traumatic dislocation of the knee. J Bone Joint Surg Br 2005;87(5):664–7.
4. Klineberg EO, Crites BM, Flinn WR, et al. The role of arteriography in assessing popliteal artery injury in knee dislocations. J Trauma 2004;56(4):786–90.

5. Mills WJ, Barei DP, McNair P. The value of the ankle-brachial index for diagnosing arterial injury after knee dislocation: a prospective study. J Trauma 2004;56(6): 1261–5.

6. James EW, Williams BT, LaPrade RF. Stress radiography for the diagnosis of knee ligament injuries: a systematic review. Clin Orthop Relat Res 2014;472(9): 2644–57.

7. Kane PW, DePhillipo NN, Cinque ME, et al. Increased accuracy of varus stress radiographs versus magnetic resonance imaging in diagnosing fibular collateral ligament grade III tears. Arthroscopy 2018;34(7):2230–5.

8. Mackay GM, Blyth MJ, Anthony I, et al. A review of ligament augmentation with the InternalBrace™: the surgical principle is described for the lateral ankle ligament and ACL repair in particular, and a comprehensive review of other surgical applications and techniques is presented [Review]. Surg Technol Int 2015;26: 239–55.

9. van Eck CF, Limpisvasti O, ElAttrache NS. Is there a role for internal bracing and repair of the anterior cruciate ligament? A systematic literature review. Am J Sports Med 2018;46(9):2291–8.

10. Fisher MB, Liang R, Jung HJ, et al. Potential of healing a transected anterior cruciate ligament with genetically modified extracellular matrix bioscaffolds in a goat model. Knee Surg Sports Traumatol Arthrosc 2012;20(7):1357–65.

11. Wilson WT, Hopper GP, Byrne PA, et al. Anterior cruciate ligament repair with internal brace ligament augmentation. Surg Technol Int 2016;29:273–8.

12. Smith JO, Yasen SK, Palmer HC, et al. Paediatric ACL repair reinforced with temporary internal bracing. Knee Surg Sports Traumatol Arthrosc 2016;24(6): 1845–51.

13. Eggli S, Röder C, Perler G, et al. Five year results of the first ten ACL patients treated with dynamic intraligamentary stabilisation. BMC Musculoskelet Disord 2016;17:105.

14. Smith PA, Bley JA. Allograft anterior cruciate ligament reconstruction utilizing internal brace augmentation. Arthrosc Tech 2016;5(5):e1143–7.

15. Bachmaier S, Smith PA, Bley J, et al. Independent suture tape reinforcement of small and standard diameter grafts for anterior cruciate ligament reconstruction: a biomechanical full construct model. Arthroscopy 2018;34(2):490–9.

16. Aboalata M, Elazab A, Halawa A, et al. The crossing internal suture augmentation technique to protect the all - inside anterior cruciateligament reconstruction graft. Arthrosc Tech 2017;6(6):e2235–40.

17. Aboalata M, Elazab A, Halawa A, et al. Internal suture augmentation technique to protect the anterior cruciate ligament reconstruction graft. Arthrosc Tech 2017; 6(5):e1633–8.

18. Wilson AJ, Yasen SK, Nancoo T, et al. Anatomic all-inside anterior cruciate ligament reconstruction using the translateral technique. Arthrosc Tech 2013;2(2): e99–104.

19. Lubowitz JH, Ahmad CS, Anderson K. All-inside anterior cruciate ligament graft-link technique: second-generation, no-incision anterior cruciate ligament reconstruction. Arthroscopy 2011;27(5):717–27.

20. Gilmer BB, Crall T, DeLong J, et al. Biomechanical analysis of internal bracing for treatment of medial knee injuries. Orthopedics 2016;39(3):e532–7.

21. LaPrade RF, Wijdicks CA. Surgical technique: development of an anatomic medial knee reconstruction. Clin Orthop Relat Res 2012;470(3):806–14.

22. Lubowitz JH, MacKay G, Gilmer B. Knee medial collateral ligament and postero-medial corner anatomic repair with internal bracing. Arthrosc Tech 2014;3(4): e505–8.

23. van der List JP, DiFelice GS. Primary repair of the medial collateral ligament with internal bracing. Arthrosc Tech 2017;6(4):e933–7.

24. Kovachevich R, Shah JP, Arens AM, et al. Operative management of the medial collateral ligament in the multi-ligament injured knee: an evidence-based system-atic review. Knee Surg Sports Traumatol Arthrosc 2009;17(7):823–9.

25. Hanley JM, Anthony CA, DeMik D, et al. Patient-reported outcomes after multili-gament knee injury: MCL repair versus reconstruction. Orthop J Sports Med 2017;5(3). 2325967117694818.

26. Stannard JP, Brown SL, Farris RC, et al. The posterolateral corner of the knee: repair versus reconstruction. Am J Sports Med 2005;33(6):881–8.

27. Levy BA, Dajani KA, Morgan JA, et al. Repair versus reconstruction of the fibular collateral ligament and posterolateral corner in the multiligament-injured knee. Am J Sports Med 2010;38(4):804–9.

28. Tardy N, Boisrenoult P, Teissier P, et al. Clinical outcomes after multiligament injured knees: medial versus lateral reconstructions. Knee Surg Sports Traumatol Arthrosc 2017;25(2):524–31.

29. Fanelli GC, Edson CJ. Arthroscopically assisted combined anterior and posterior cruciate ligament reconstruction in the multiple ligament injured knee: 2- to 10-year follow-up. Arthroscopy 2002;18(7):703–14.

30. Geeslin AG, LaPrade RF. Outcomes of treatment of acute grade-III isolated and combined posterolateral knee injuries: a prospective case series and surgical technique. J Bone Joint Surg Am 2011;93(18):1672–83.

31. Geeslin AG, Moulton SG, LaPrade RF. A systematic review of the outcomes of posterolateral corner knee injuries, part 1: surgical treatment of acute injuries. Am J Sports Med 2016;44(5):1336–42.

32. Nancoo TJ, Lord B, Yasen SK, et al. Transmedial all-inside posterior cruciate lig-ament reconstruction using a reinforced tibial inlay graft. Arthrosc Tech 2013;2(4): e381–8.

33. Yasen SK, Borton ZM, Britton EM, et al. Transmedial all-inside trilink posterior cru-ciate ligament reconstruction. Arthrosc Tech 2017;6(5):e1871–7.

34. Trasolini NA, Rick Hatch GF 3rd. Suture augmentation: an alternative to recon-struction for incomplete posterior cruciate ligament injuries in the multiple ligament-injured knee. Arthrosc Tech 2018;7(3):e239–43.

35. Frosch KH, Preiss A, Heider S, et al. Primary ligament sutures as a treatment op-tion of knee dislocations: a meta-analysis. Knee Surg Sports Traumatol Arthrosc 2013;21(7):1502–9.

36. Heitmann M, Gerau M, Hötzel J, et al. Ligament bracing–augmented primary su-ture repair in multiligamentous kneeinjuries. Oper Orthop Traumatol 2014;26(1): 19–29 [in German].

37. Levy BA, Dajani KA, Whelan DB, et al. Decision making in the multiligament-injured knee: an evidence-based systematic review. Arthroscopy 2009;25(4): 430–8.

38. Schenck RC Jr, Hunter RE, Ostrum RF, et al. Knee dislocations. Instr Course Lect 1999;48:515–22.

All-inside Posterior Cruciate Ligament Reconstruction
Surgical Technique and Outcome

Benjamin Freychet, MD[a,b], Vishal S. Desai, BS[a,b],
Thomas L. Sanders, MD[a,b], Nicholas I. Kennedy, MD[a,b],
Aaron J. Krych, MD[a,b], Michael J. Stuart, MD[a,b],
Bruce A. Levy, MD[a,b,*]

KEYWORDS

- Posterior cruciate ligament deficiency • Posterior cruciate ligament reconstruction
- All-inside technique • Bone preservation • Tunnel convergence
- Sequential graft tensioning

KEY POINTS

- All-inside ACL technique reconstruction reported good or excellent outcomes.
- All-inside technique has the potential to conserve bone and decrease the risk of tunnel convergence in the setting of multi-ligament knee surgery.
- Adjustable loop fixation on both sides of the graft has been reported to allow more optimal graft tensioning.

INTRODUCTION

Despite advances in knowledge about posterior cruciate ligament (PCL) anatomy and function, the optimal surgical approach, graft choice, and reconstruction technique remain controversial. Double-bundle (DB), single-bundle (SB), transtibial, and tibial inlay techniques have been described for PCL reconstruction (PCLR) and all are associated with successful clinical outcomes.[1–9] Additional studies have demonstrated satisfactory subjective and objective clinical outcomes after PCLR using either autograft or allograft tissue.[10,11]

Numerous studies comparing SB versus DB reconstruction found no difference in Lysholm or International Knee Documentation Committee (IKDC) scores and no side-to-side differences in anteroposterior instability.[8,11–15] Regarding transtibial versus tibial inlay PCLR, McAllister and colleagues[16] demonstrated no difference

---

[a] Department of Orthopedic Surgery, Mayo Clinic, 200 First Street Southwest, Rochester, MN 55905, USA; [b] Department of Sports Medicine, Mayo Clinic, 200 First Street Southwest, Rochester, MN 55905, USA
* Corresponding author.
E-mail address: Levy.Bruce@mayo.edu

Clin Sports Med 38 (2019) 285–295
https://doi.org/10.1016/j.csm.2018.11.005
0278-5919/19/© 2018 Elsevier Inc. All rights reserved.

between the 2 techniques in biomechanical studies and both surgical techniques have demonstrated satisfactory clinical and functional results.[7–9]

Recently, several investigators have described the all-inside PCLR technique, which relies on adjustable-loop cortical fixation and creating a tibia bone socket instead of a full-length tibia bone tunnel. This new technique has the potential to conserve bone and decrease the risk of tunnel convergence in the setting of multiligament knee surgery. Additionally, adjustable-loop fixation on both sides of the graft has been reported to allow more optimal graft tensioning.[17–20]

Currently, there are no studies reporting clinical knee outcome after all-inside PCLR. The purpose of this study was to evaluate subjective and objective knee outcomes after all-inside PCLR at 2 years' follow-up. The study hypothesis was that all-inside PCLR would result in similar knee functional outcomes compared with previously described PCLR techniques.

METHODS

Approval from the Institutional Review Board, No. 15-000601, was granted prior to commencement of this study. The first all-inside PCLR was performed in October 2012. Therefore, the medical records were queried in the authors' prospective multiligament knee injury (MLKI) database for patients who had undergone primary all-inside PCLR using soft tissue allograft between October 2012 and June 2017. Patients required at least 3 months of clinical examination follow-up and at least 12 months of patient-reported outcomes. All patients had undergone preoperative assessment with clinical examination and stress radiographs as well as MRI. Patient demographics, injury history, and surgical details were extracted from the electronic medical record. Documented physical examination findings, including ligamentous stability examination, were recorded from clinic and operative notes. Preoperative and postoperative bilateral comparison stress radiography using kneeling stress views became systematically used starting in January 2014 and were available postoperatively on 14 of the 32 patients. Patients with isolated PCL injuries were denoted as such and those with multiligament involvement were assigned knee dislocation (KD) grades as defined by the Schenck classification (see **Table 3**).[21] The authors' institution uses a prospective collection system of patient-reported outcomes, which was used to record Lysholm, IKDC, and Tegner activity level scale scores. All ligament surgeries were performed in a simultaneous fashion.

Concomitant injuries, ligament reconstructions, and other procedures performed at the time of all-inside PCLR are shown below (**Tables 1–3**). Surgical interval was categorized as follows: acute (<3 weeks from injury), semiacute (3–6 weeks from injury), and delayed (>6 weeks from injury).[22]

Surgical Technique

The technique used in this study has been previously described.[18]

Table 1	
Concomitant ligamentous reconstructions at time of all-inside posterior cruciate ligament reconstruction	
ACL reconstruction	18
Medial collateral ligament reconstruction	10
FCL and PLC reconstruction	15

Table 2
Concomitant injuries at time of all-inside posterior cruciate ligament reconstruction

Cartilage injury	11
Meniscus injury	14
Peroneal nerve injury	10
Popliteal artery injury	6

Patient preparation and positioning

An examination under anesthesia with fluoroscopic stress examination comparing side-to-side differences is performed prior to patient positioning. A tourniquet is applied (for emergent purposes) but generally is not used. Standard positioning based on surgeon preference with the use of leg holders is performed.

Approach

Standard superomedial, anterolateral, and anteromedial (AM) portals and an accessory low AM portal are established and routine diagnostic arthroscopy is completed. All meniscus and cartilage lesions are treated at this time. A posteromedial portal is then established, and a 30° arthroscope is used initially. The posteromedial portal is used to clear the PCL tibial footprint, with care taken to release the midline septum to allow the neurovascular bundle to retract posteriorly. Viewing through either the high AM or low AM portal allows best visualization of the tibial footprint at this point. The authors then recommend switching to a 70° arthroscope, which allows excellent visualization of the entire PCL facet as well as the mammillary bodies. The combination of a shaver (Stryker, Kalamazoo, Michigan) and radiofrequency device (Arthro-Care, Austin, Texas) is used to clear the PCL footprint between the mammillary bodies and distally all the way to the base of the PCL facet past the champagne drop-off where the popliteus muscle belly comes into view.

Tibial socket preparation

The PCL anatomic contoured guide (Arthrex, Naples, Florida), designed to wrap around the entire PCL facet, is introduced through the low AM portal while the surgeon is viewing from the AL portal. The guide fits anatomically between the mammillary bodies and hooks the posterior tibia at the base of the PCL facet (**Fig. 1**). Anteriorly, the guide is positioned approximately 1-cm medial to the tibial crest. The arthroscope is then placed in the posteromedial portal to allow direct visualization of the guide pin followed by the FlipCutter (Arthrex). The guide serves as a neurovascular shield during drilling. The tibial socket is reamed to a depth of 35 mm. A FiberStick (Arthrex) is used

Table 3
Knee dislocation classification

PCL only	5
KD grade 1	8
KD grade 2	3
KD grade 3 medial	4
KD grade 3 lateral	5
KD grade 4	0
KD grade 5	7
TOTAL	32

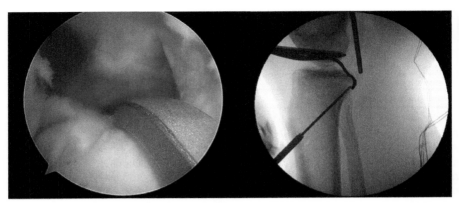

Fig. 1. Intraoperative views of PCL guide placement during all-inside PCLR. Intra-articular view (*left*). Peroperative X-ray view (*right*).

to establish a passing suture into the tibial socket. This completes the preparation of the tibial socket.

Femoral socket preparation

A low AL portal is created with a spinal needle for femoral socket creation. The low-profile reamer (Arthrex) itself or an inside-out guide is positioned at the center of the anterolateral bundle (ALB) femoral footprint just off the medial femoral condyle articular cartilage. A 2.4-mm guide pin (Arthrex) is inserted and the low-profile reamer drilled to a depth of 25 mm. A spade-tip pin (Arthrex) is then used to measure the interosseous length and insert a passing suture into the femoral socket. A PassPort cannula (Arthrex) in the low AL portal prevents a soft tissue bridge when retrieving the femoral and tibial passing sutures. The femoral side of the graft is marked at the measured interosseous length.

Graft preparation

A soft tissue allograft with a minimum length of 340 mm is recommended to allow quadrupling of the allograft to 90 mm, which provides at least 20 mm in the femoral and tibial sockets. The femoral end is looped over the TightRope RT (Arthrex) and the tibial end over a TightRope ABS (Arthrex) loop. Each graft end is sutured approximately 2 cm from its corresponding loop. A graft thickness of 10 mm to 12 mm is desired depending on the size of the patient (**Fig. 2**).

In this study, 16 of the all-inside PCLRs were performed using a peroneus longus allograft, 15 using a tibialis anterior allograft, and 1 using a semitendinosus allograft, and the mean graft diameter was 11.0 mm (SD 0.80 mm).

Graft passage and fixation

The tibial side of the graft is passed first and pulled as deep as possible into the tibial socket, which facilitates easier passage of the femoral end. A suture-grasping instrument is used to hold constant tension while the TightRope is pulled into the femoral socket. The TightRope button can be directly visualized as it passes the femoral cortex, and the marked osseous length acts as a second check before it is flipped. The TightRope is then used to dock the femoral end of the graft in its corresponding socket. The ABS button (Arthrex) is attached to the tibial TightRope, and the tibial end of the graft is secured on the AM tibia. The knee is flexed and extended to remove creep from the graft. Final tensioning is performed with the knee flexed to 90° with an

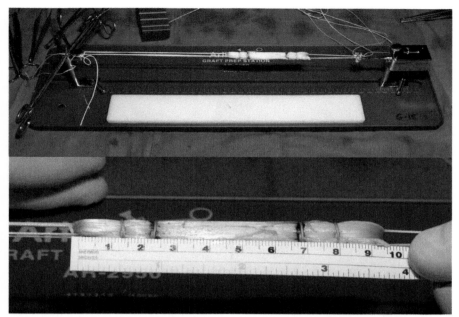

Fig. 2. Graft preparation using a quadrupled tibialis anterior allograft, approximately 90-mm long and 10-mm to 12-mm thick. Two loop stitches are placed on each end of the graft.

anterior drawer with both tibial and femoral TightRope tensioning and retensioning. Backup fixation with a 5.5-mm SwiveLock (Arthrex) may be used (**Figs. 3** and **4**).

Rehabilitation Protocol

The postoperative rehabilitation program is patterned after the protocol developed by Edson and Fanelli.[23,24] The authors use a PCL brace after surgery to minimize gravitational forces on the tibia while the patient is supine. The brace is locked in extension during ambulation, and the patient remains partially weight bearing with crutches for the first 6 weeks. The patient is allowed to start prone, passive knee flexion to 90 immediately. After 6 weeks, progressive weight bearing as tolerated is allowed with crutches and the brace unlocked. Closed kinetic chain exercises, range of motion, core strengthening, and attainment of a normal gait pattern are the goals from 6 weeks to 12 weeks postoperatively. Isolated hamstring exercises are not allowed for the first 4 months (isolated PCLR) or 6 months (PCLR and posterolateral corner reconstruction), and the brace is worn full time for the first year.

Statistical Analysis

Descriptive statistics, including mean, median, SD, and range, were used to assess the available demographic data, injury history, and surgical details for the patient cohort. Univariate analysis, including statistical hypothesis testing, was used as appropriate. Sample size was taken into account for all calculations. The Wilcoxon rank sum test was used to analyze any correlation between outcomes scores and preoperative patient factors, such as age, neurovascular involvement, meniscus and cartilage injury, and KD grade, as well as to assess for any significant difference between preinjury and postoperative Tegner scores. Comparisons of preoperative and postoperative scores were conducted using a matched-pair analysis. All statistical

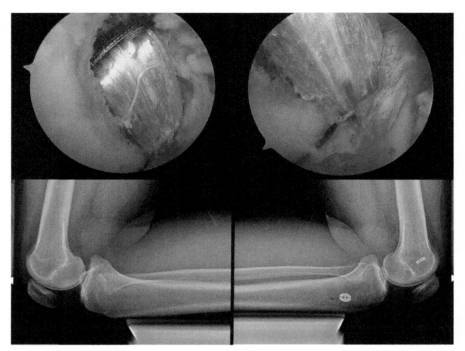

Fig. 3. Arthroscopic views of an isolated PCLR and postoperative comparison stress views demonstrating 0-mm side-to-side difference. Arthroscopic views (*Top left and right*). Stress views (*Bottom left and right*).

analysis was performed using Microsoft Excel version 14.0 (Redmond, Washington) and JMP version 13.0 (Cary, North Carolina).

RESULTS

A total of 32 patients (32 knees) (23 men and 9 women) with a mean age of 27 (SD 10.8) and mean follow-up of 24.0 months (SD 15.9; range 12.0–65.3) met inclusion criteria. Median duration from injury to reconstruction was 169 days (range 18–5109); 28 patients underwent delayed surgery, 2 received acute surgery, and 2 patients underwent semiacute surgery.

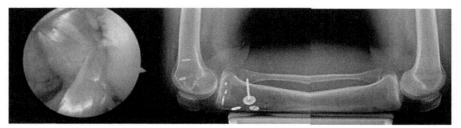

Fig. 4. Arthroscopic view of a combined ACL-PCL–medial collateral ligament reconstruction and postoperative comparison stress views demonstrating 1.2-mm side-to-side difference. Intra articular arthroscopic view (*left*). Comparative stress view (*right*).

Physical examination findings were measured at final follow-up at a mean of 16.0 months (SD 11.1). Mean extension was 0.4° (SD 1.8; range −5° to 5°) and mean flexion was 124° (SD 12.2; range 90°–140°). Ligament stability testing data at preoperative examination and final follow-up are shown below in **Tables 4** and **5**. Mean side-to-side difference on kneeling stress radiographs was +1.1 mm (see **Figs. 3** and **4**).

Patient-reported outcomes data at a mean of 24.1 months (range 12.0–65.3 months) is shown in **Table 6**.

There were no significant differences between patients who suffered either vascular or peroneal nerve damage at the time of initial injury and those without Lysholm (86.1 vs 84.6; $P = .697$), IKDC (85.4 vs 82.1; $P = .935$), and Tegner (7.0 vs 6.3; $P = .127$) scores. Patients with meniscus and/or chondral injuries at the time of PCLR did not demonstrate any significantly worse outcomes at follow-up compared with patients without meniscus or cartilage injury. Outcomes in patients who were greater than 30 years versus less than or equal to 30 years of age at the time of PCLR did not significantly differ (Lysholm 85.7 vs 84.9, $P = .512$; IKDC 80.6 vs 84.1, $P = .257$; and Tegner 6.5 vs 6.5, $P = .899$). There was no significant difference in mean postoperative Tegner activity score (7.0) compared with the mean preinjury value (6.6) ($P = .054$). There were no significant difference outcomes scores when stratified by KD grade (**Fig. 5**).

Rupture of the PCL graft (failure) was not seen in any of the 32 cases. One patient required manipulation and arthroscopic lysis of adhesions and 1 patient developed partial wound dehiscence, which required wound irrigation and closure without administration of antibiotics. There were no cases of residual laxity requiring revision surgery, iatrogenic vascular injury, or painful hardware.

DISCUSSION

The results of this study demonstrate that the all-inside PCLR technique results in satisfactory subjective and objective knee function. Neither age nor gender nor KD grade nor meniscus or cartilage injury nor peroneal or vascular injury was associated with poor subjective outcomes. Although the authors did not directly compare the all-inside technique with DB or tibial inlay PCLR techniques, this study demonstrates similar clinical outcomes as other PCLR techniques.[1–9]

The all-inside technique is bone conserving and decreases the risk of tunnel convergence in the setting of multiligament knee surgery.[17–20] The use of adjustable-loop fixation on both sides of the graft has been reported as a reliable graft fixation option without evidence of loosening after anterior cruciate ligament (ACL) reconstruction.[25,26] Noonan and colleagues[27] reported that retensioning and knot tying of the

Table 4	
Preoperative ligament stability physical examination results	
Posterior drawer examination	
Negative	0
2+	12
3+	20
Posterior sag test	
Negative	0
1+	32

Table 5 Postoperative ligament stability physical examination results	
Posterior drawer examination	
Negative	25
1+	7
Posterior sag test	
Negative	27
1+	5

adjustable-loop fixation reduced final cyclic elongation by 50% compared with a closed-loop device after ACL reconstruction.

Several investigators have reported good outcomes with SB transtibial PCLR technique.[1-3] Ahn and colleagues[1] reported a mean Lysholm score improvement from 65.8 to 92.9 with patients who underwent PCLR with preservation of PCL fibers. Sekiya and colleagues[2] reported 57% of the patients had normal/near-normal knee function, and 62% had a normal/near-normal activity level after arthroscopic PCLR in patients with isolated grade III PCL injuries. In this study, there was no association between meniscal or cartilage injury and postoperative knee scores. Similarly, a recent study with minimum 10 years of follow-up, Moatshe and colleagues[28] reported meniscal and cartilage injuries at time of surgery were not associated with the development of osteoathritis. In contrast, a recent study from the Mayo Clinic reported both articular cartilage damage and combined medial and lateral meniscus tears were predictive of inferior IKDC scores after multiligament reconstructive surgery.[29] A recent systematic review evaluating PCLR concluded that normal knee stability was not fully restored but found a significant reduction in posterior knee laxity and improved mean Lysholm knee score.[3]

In this present study, a majority of patients had combined ligament reconstructions. Mygind-Klavsen and colleagues[11] compared clinical outcomes between isolated PCL and MLKIs with a mean follow-up of 5.9 years. At 1-year follow-up, there were significant differences in Knee injury and Osteoarthritis Outcome Score (KOOS) outcome scores between the isolated PCL subgroup and the multiligament subgroup but no differences at final follow-up.[11] The mean IKDC scores at final follow-up were 63.8 in the isolated PCL group and 65.0 in the combined PCL group.[11] Spiridonov and colleagues[30] found significant improvements in both subjective (Cincinnati and IKDC) and objective outcome scores in patients with either isolated or combined ligament injuries. Owesen and colleagues[31] from the Norwegian ACL registry published 2-year follow-up data after isolated PCLR in 71 patients. They found similar incremental improvements in KOOS comparing PCL and ACL patients.[31]

The optimal timing of surgical treatment of PCL tears (isolated or with concomitant ligament injuries) remains unclear. In our study, a majority of patients (91%) had surgery greater than 6 weeks after their injury. Spiridonov and colleagues[30] reported knee function using a DB transtibial technique in isolated or combined PCL tears. They

Table 6 Mean patient-reported outcomes	
IKDC score	85.0 (SD 13.5)
Lysholm score	87.4 (SD 13.1)
Tegner score	6.6 (SD 1.0)

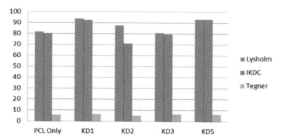

Fig. 5. Mean outcomes score by KD grade.

found no difference between acute and chronic surgery (defined as more than 6 weeks from injury) in posterior translation on stress radiographs or subjective knee scores (Cincinnati and IKDC).[30] Some studies in multiligament knee injuries have suggested that acute treatment (within 3 weeks from injury) has a significantly higher rate of arthrofibrosis and need for secondary surgery/manipulation compared with the chronic treatment (more than 3 weeks from injury).[32] Overall final range of motion in this study, however, was not found significantly different. On the contrary, 2 other recent systematic reviews found acute treatment to have significantly higher Lysholm and IKDC scores than late (chronic) treatment.[22,33] Likewise, Jiang and colleagues[34] found no statistically significant differences between acute and chronic treatment of PCL injuries. Ultimately, surgical timing is dictated by many patient-specific and knee-specific factors, including ligament disruption pattern and associated injuries.

In our study, there was no significant difference in outcome based on KD grade. Recently, Mygind-Klavsen and colleagues[11] reported outcomes after PCLR for isolated or combined PCL tears. They also found no significant difference when comparing KD grades I–II with KD grades III–IV.[11]

Peroneal nerve injury (complete or partial) and vascular injury at the time of final follow-up was also not associated with poor knee outcomes. Krych and colleagues[35] reported no difference in Lysholm or IKDC scores between patients with or without peroneal nerve injury after MLKI. With regard to vascular injuries and outcomes, Sanders and colleagues[36] recently reported a matched cohort analysis and found significantly lower knee function scores in patients with an associated popliteal artery injury requiring bypass grafting in the setting of MLKI.

Our study has several limitations, including limited sample size, lack of a control group, retrospective design, and heterogeneity of injury patterns. Despite these limitations, PCLR is an infrequent surgical procedure and this study cohort is relatively large, considering the incidence of PCL injury. Kneeling stress radiographs were only available in 14 of 32 patients. As a tertiary-care center, many patients travel for their surgical procedure and had postoperative follow-up locally. The strengths of this study include prospective database collection and a standardized surgical technique and rehabilitation protocol.

SUMMARY

The authors' series using the all-inside, SB PCLR demonstrated satisfactory clinical and functional outcomes comparable with previous other PCLR techniques. The advantages of this technique include bone preservation (using sockets instead of full tunnels), minimizing risk of tunnel convergence (in combined/multiligament knee surgery), and allowing for sequential graft tensioning.

REFERENCES

1. Ahn JH, Yang HS, Jeong WK, et al. Arthroscopic transtibial posterior cruciate ligament reconstruction with preservation of posterior cruciate ligament fibers: clinical results of minimum 2year follow-up. Am J Sports Med 2006;34(2):194–204.
2. Sekiya JK, West RV, Ong BC, et al. Clinical outcomes after isolated arthroscopic single-bundle posterior cruciate ligament reconstruction. Arthroscopy 2005; 21(9):1042–50.
3. Kim Y-M, Lee CA, Matava MJ. Clinical results of arthroscopic single-bundle transtibial posterior cruciate ligament reconstruction: a systematic review. Am J Sports Med 2011;39(2):425–34.
4. Milles JL, Nuelle CW, Pfeiffer F, et al. Biomechanical comparison: single-bundle versus double-bundle posterior cruciate ligament reconstruction techniques. J Knee Surg 2017;30(04):347–51.
5. Li Y, Li J, Wang J, et al. Comparison of single-bundle and double-bundle isolated posterior cruciate ligament reconstruction with allograft: a prospective, randomized study. Arthroscopy 2014;30(6):695–700.
6. Yoon KH, Bae DK, Song SJ, et al. A prospective randomized study comparing arthroscopic single-bundle and double-bundle posterior cruciate ligament reconstructions preserving remnant fibers. Am J Sports Med 2011;39(3):474–80.
7. May JH, Gillette BP, Morgan JA, et al. Transtibial versus inlay posterior cruciate ligament reconstruction: an evidence-based systematic review. J Knee Surg 2010;23(02):073–80.
8. Shin Y-S, Kim H-J, Lee D-H. No clinically important difference in knee scores or instability between transtibial and inlay techniques for PCL reconstruction: a systematic review. Clin Orthop Relat Res 2017;475(4):1239–48.
9. Song E-K, Park H-W, Ahn Y-S, et al. Transtibial versus tibial inlay techniques for posterior cruciate ligament reconstruction: long-term follow-up study. Am J Sports Med 2014;42(12):2964–71.
10. Hudgens JL, Gillette BP, Krych AJ, et al. Allograft versus autograft in posterior cruciate ligament reconstruction: an evidence-based systematic review. J Knee Surg 2013;26(02):109–16.
11. Mygind-Klavsen B, Nielsen TG, Lind MC. Outcomes after posterior cruciate ligament (PCL) reconstruction in patients with isolated and combined PCL tears. Orthopaedic J Sports Med 2017;5(4). 2325967117700077.
12. Deie M, Adachi N, Nakamae A, et al. Evaluation of single-bundle versus double-bundle PCL reconstructions with more than 10-year follow-up. ScientificWorldJournal 2015;2015:751465.
13. Fanelli GC, Beck JD, Edson CJ. Single compared to double-bundle PCL reconstruction using allograft tissue. J Knee Surg 2012;25(01):059–64.
14. Qi Y-S, Wang H-J, Wang S-J, et al. A systematic review of double-bundle versus single-bundle posterior cruciate ligament reconstruction. BMC Musculoskelet Disord 2016;17(1):45.
15. Kohen RB, Sekiya JK. Single-bundle versus double-bundle posterior cruciate ligament reconstruction. Arthroscopy 2009;25(12):1470–7.
16. McAllister DR, Markolf KL, Oakes DA, et al. A biomechanical comparison of tibial inlay and tibial tunnel posterior cruciate ligament reconstruction techniques: graft pretension and knee laxity. Am J Sports Med 2002;30(3):312–7.
17. Adler GG. All-inside posterior cruciate ligament reconstruction with a GraftLink. Arthrosc Tech 2013;2(2):e111–5.

18. Prince MR, Stuart MJ, King AH, et al. All-inside posterior cruciate ligament reconstruction: GraftLink technique. Arthrosc Tech 2015;4(5):e619–24.
19. Vasdev A, Rajgopal A, Gupta H, et al. Arthroscopic all-inside posterior cruciate ligament reconstruction: overcoming the "killer turn". Arthrosc Tech 2016;5(3):e501–6.
20. Brossard P, Boutsiadis A, Panisset J-C, et al. Adjustable button devices for all-arthroscopic posterior cruciate ligament reconstruction using the hamstrings tendons and the "forgotten" transseptal approach. Arthrosc Tech 2017;6(4):e979–85.
21. Schenck RC. Classification of knee dislocations. The multiple ligament injured knee. New York: Springer; 2004. p. 37–49.
22. Levy BA, Dajani KA, Whelan DB, et al. Decision making in the multiligament-injured knee: an evidence-based systematic review. Arthroscopy 2009;25(4):430–8.
23. Edson CJ. Postoperative rehabilitation of the multiligament-reconstructed knee. Sports Med Arthrosc Rev 2001;9(3):247–54.
24. Edson CJ, Fanelli GC, Beck JD. Rehabilitation after multiple-ligament reconstruction of the knee. Sports Med Arthrosc Rev 2011;19(2):162–6.
25. Boyle MJ, Vovos TJ, Walker CG, et al. Does adjustable-loop femoral cortical suspension loosen after anterior cruciate ligament reconstruction? A retrospective comparative study. Knee 2015;22(4):304–8.
26. Nye DD, Mitchell WR, Liu W, et al. Biomechanical comparison of fixed-loop and adjustable-loop cortical suspensory devices for metaphyseal femoral-sided soft tissue graft fixation in anatomic anterior cruciate ligament reconstruction using a porcine model. Arthroscopy 2017;33(6):1225–32.e1.
27. Noonan BC, Dines JS, Allen AA, et al. Biomechanical evaluation of an adjustable loop suspensory anterior cruciate ligament reconstruction fixation device: the value of retensioning and knot tying. Arthroscopy 2016;32(10):2050–9.
28. Moatshe G, Dornan GJ, Ludvigsen T, et al. High prevalence of knee osteoarthritis at a minimum 10-year follow-up after knee dislocation surgery. Knee Surg Sports Traumatol Arthrosc 2017;25(12):3914–22.
29. King AH, Krych AJ, Prince MR, et al. Are meniscal tears and articular cartilage injury predictive of inferior patient outcome after surgical reconstruction for the dislocated knee? Knee Surg Sports Traumatol Arthrosc 2015;23(10):3008–11.
30. Spiridonov SI, Slinkard NJ, LaPrade RF. Isolated and combined grade-III posterior cruciate ligament tears treated with double-bundle reconstruction with use of endoscopically placed femoral tunnels and grafts: operative technique and clinical outcomes. J Bone Joint Surg Am 2011;93(19):1773–80.
31. Owesen C, Sivertsen EA, Engebretsen L, et al. Patients with isolated PCL injuries improve from surgery as much as patients with ACL injuries after 2 years. Orthopaedic J Sports Med 2015;3(8). 2325967115599539.
32. Mook WR, Miller MD, Diduch DR, et al. Multiple-ligament knee injuries: a systematic review of the timing of operative intervention and postoperative rehabilitation. J Bone Joint Surg Am 2009;91(12):2946–57.
33. Hohmann E, Glatt V, Tetsworth K. Early or delayed reconstruction in multiligament knee injuries: a systematic review and meta-analysis. Knee 2017;24(5):909–16.
34. Jiang W, Yao J, He Y, et al. The timing of surgical treatment of knee dislocations: a systematic review. Knee Surg Sports Traumatol Arthrosc 2015;23(10):3108–13.
35. Krych AJ, Giuseffi SA, Kuzma SA, et al. Is peroneal nerve injury associated with worse function after knee dislocation? Clin Orthop Relat Res 2014;472(9):2630–6.
36. Sanders TL, Johnson NR, Levy NM, et al. Effect of vascular injury on functional outcome in knees with multi-ligament injury: a matched-cohort analysis. J Bone Joint Surg Am 2017;99(18):1565–71.

Osteotomies in the Multiple Ligament Injured Knee

When Is It Necessary?

Niv Marom, MD[a], Norimasa Nakamura, MD, PhD[b],
Robert G. Marx, MD[a],*, Michael J. Stuart, MD[c]

KEYWORDS

- Multiple ligament-injured knee • Osteotomy • Posterior tibial slope • Varus thrust
- Triple varus • Coronal malalignment • Opening wedge osteotomy
- Closing wedge osteotomy

KEY POINTS

- In the setting of the unstable and malaligned knee, isolated reconstructive ligament procedures are prone to failure if the limb is not realigned.
- Literature supports osteotomy in addition to ligament reconstructive procedures in knees with complex double/triple varus injury patterns and have shown good outcomes after combined or staged procedures.
- Corrective osteotomies of the tibial slope, either in isolation or combined with coronal realignment, are an additional important tool that addresses and treats anterior-posterior instability.
- In revisions of failed multiple ligament reconstruction surgery, a corrective osteotomy should be considered with any coronal malalignment greater than 5°.
- In some unstable and malaligned multiple ligament injured knees, corrective osteotomies may provide sufficient stability, functionality, and pain reduction, and additional soft tissues procedures may be unnecessary.

INTRODUCTION

The multiple ligament-injured knee is often associated with additional intra- and extra-articular injuries. Surgical repair and reconstruction of the involved ligaments are frequently discussed in the literature; however, osteotomy to correct limb malalignment may be just as important to obtaining a good outcome.

Veltri and Warren[1] outlined the role of osteotomy in the unstable, malaligned knee in the coronal plane with or without a varus thrust gait. They showed that any

[a] Hospital for Special Surgery, 535 East 70th Street, New York, NY 10021, USA; [b] Institute for Medical Science in Sports, Osaka Health Science University, 1-9-27 Tenma, Kita-ku, Osaka City, Osaka 530-0043, Japan; [c] Mayo Clinic, 201 West Center Street, Rochester, MN 55902, USA
* Corresponding author.
E-mail address: marxr@hss.edu

Clin Sports Med 38 (2019) 297–304
https://doi.org/10.1016/j.csm.2018.11.003
0278-5919/19/© 2018 Elsevier Inc. All rights reserved.

reconstructive procedure is prone to failure if the limb is not realigned because of chronic repetitive overload on the reconstructed tissue secondary to the malalignment.

This article will discuss the role of osteotomy in the treatment of the multiple ligament-injured knee.

CORONAL MALALIGNMENT
The Varus Knee

Varus malalignment represents several clinical conditions with distinct characteristics. Primary or single varus refers to the osseous (tibiofemoral) varus alignment with or without medial compartment narrowing secondary to damaged medial meniscus and/or articular cartilage. The transfer of the weight-bearing line into the medial compartment results in higher compressive loads, increased tensile forces, and excessive laxity of the lateral capsuloligamentous structures, all of which represent a double varus knee. The development of a double varus knee leads to further degeneration of the articular cartilage. Additional compromise of the posterolateral structures can occur over time, resulting in a varus/recurvatum or triple varus knee.[2] Varus thrust, often seen in double or triple varus conditions, refers to a dynamic alignment abnormality. The thrust is identified by an abrupt worsening of varus during the weight-bearing phase of gait, which corrects during the nonweight=bearing (swing) phase.[3,4]

Varus malalignment, with or without thrust, has been implicated as a potential cause for increased anterior cruciate ligament (ACL) strain and a potential risk factor for ACL reconstruction failure.[4–6] Additionally, cadaveric studies have shown that the application of a varus torque to the extended knee results higher tension forces within the ACL. Noyes and colleagues[7] recommended osteotomy in addition to ligament reconstructive procedures in knees with complex double and triple varus injury patterns and showed good outcomes after combined or staged procedures.

Acute injury to the posterolateral complex in combination with ACL injury and preexisting varus alignment simulates a triple varus knee. The addition of a posterior cruciate ligament (PCL) injury can augment the hyperextension deformity, and combined ACL, PCL, and posterolateral corner injuries can further magnify hyperextension, varus and external rotational deformities.[8] Addressing only the soft tissues when treating these complex injuries will result high rates of failures.[9] A recent systematic review by Tischer and colleagues[10] provided clinical evidence to support osseous malalignment as a contributing factor to failure of knee ligament surgery. These authors recommended limb realignment surgery in selected cases to improve function and stability, especially with posterolateral corner insufficiency.

Phisitkul and colleagues[11] suggested that osteotomy is indicated in patients with varus thrust gait and posterolateral laxity. They recommended an opening wedge, valgus-producing, proximal tibial osteotomy to produce a multi-planar correction with better intraoperative adjustment and avoidance of the proximal tibiofibular joint and peroneal nerve. Disadvantages of this technique include possible need for bone graft and difficulty in correcting severe deformities. The lateral closing wedge valgus-producing proximal tibial osteotomy remains an option and provides a stable construct with good bone apposition. However, a closing wedge can decrease posterior tibial slope, which may negatively affect a PCL-deficient knee. In addition, tibial shortening decreases the distance between the tibial plateau and tibial tuberosity, increases lateral collateral ligament laxity, and may have an unfavorable impact on future conversion to total knee arthroplasty.[8]

Alignment correction, regardless of technique, transfers the weight-bearing line (center of the femoral head to center of the talus) to the 62.5% position on the tibial plateau when measured from medial to lateral.[8]

In scenarios in which instability is combined with clear degenerative changes in the overloaded compartment, realignment procedures are indicated for additional reasons, as they can redistribute the joint forces and decrease symptoms related to osteoarthritis.[6] A medial opening wedge proximal tibial osteotomy in the varus knee will produce lower medial compartment pressures only after subsequent release of the distal medial collateral ligament (MCL).[12]

The Valgus Knee

A severe valgus-aligned limb with excessive tensile forces on the medial side of the knee can produce a triple valgus variant. This combination of severe osseous valgus malalignment, medial soft tissue laxity, and medial joint space opening leads to eventual additional rotatory instability with further compromise of the posteromedial structures.

Phisitkul and colleagues[11] previously defined excessive valgus deformity as a weight-bearing line that falls lateral to the lateral tibial spine on a single- or double-leg weight-bearing radiograph.

The preferred way to treat these complex valgus deformities with symptoms of instability, pain, and possible medial thrust is a distal femoral lateral opening wedge or medial closing wedge osteotomy. Soft tissue procedures performed in isolation are not the proper treatment option in these circumstances.[8,13,14] Biomechanically, it has been shown that lateral opening wedge distal femoral osteotomy decreased medial knee opening when medial structures were sectioned.[14]

The lateral opening wedge osteotomy (**Figs. 1** and **2**) is becoming more popular, mainly because of the simple surgical exposure, single bone cut, and possibly more accurate correction. However, medial closing wedge osteotomy is preferred for larger corrections (>17.5°), earlier weight bearing, and if the patient has predisposing factors for delayed healing.[15]

In cases in which the osseous malaligned multiple injured knee presents with additional intra-articulator pathologies that require treatment, such as cartilage restoration or meniscal transplantation, a realignment procedure should be considered, not only for stability purposes, but also for redistribution of joint forces to protect these tissues.[16,17]

SAGITTAL MALALIGNMENT
Posterior Tibial Slope

Malalignment in the sagittal plane influences knee stability in the setting of ligamentous injury, especially with cruciate ligament rupture.[8,11,18,19] Normal posterior tibial slope values are between 9° to 11° medially and 6° to 8° laterally with a large amount of variation. Posterior tibial slope greater than 13° has been considered excessive.[20] Increased posterior tibial slope allows increased anterior tibial translation owing to the tendency of the femur to slide posteriorly. Increased anterior tibial slope allows increased posterior tibial translation owing to the tendency of the femur to slide anteriorly. In an ACL-deficient knee, anterior tibial translation is magnified by increased posterior slope and reduced with decreased posterior slope. In a PCL-deficient knee, posterior tibial translation is magnified by increased anterior slope and reduced with decreased anterior slope.

The medial opening wedge, valgus-producing, proximal tibial osteotomy can produce combined biplanar, coronal, and sagittal realignment, depending on the location

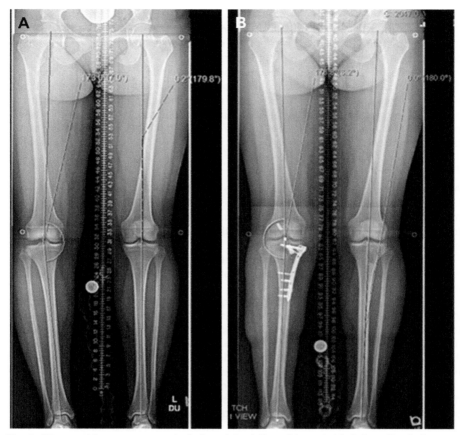

Fig. 1. 20-year-old woman presented after right ACL and lateral side injury. Physical exam-ination revealed varus and valgus thrust gait and anterior knee instability. (*A*) AP alignment radiograph showing 7° of varus on the right knee compares to no varus on the left. (*B*) AP alignment radiograph after a proximal medial opening wedge osteotomy and ACL recon-struction. Varus thrust gait was eliminated after surgery.

of the intact cortical hinge and the degree of anterior or posterior opening. A more posterolateral hinge will result in a larger change and increase in posterior tibial slope, whereas lateral cortical hinge will result in mainly coronal realignment and minimal sagittal slope change.[8,21] Increased posterior tibial opening will decrease posterior tibial slope, and increased anterior opening will increase slope.

Other osteotomies directed at changing sagittal alignment are anterior closing wedge proximal tibial osteotomy to reduce the posterior tibial slope in the setting of ACL defi-ciency (**Fig. 3**) and anterior opening wedge proximal tibial osteotomy to increase the posterior tibial slope in the setting of genu recurvatum and PCL deficiency (**Fig. 4**).

Corrective osteotomies of the tibial slope, either in isolation or combined with cor-onal realignment, are another important tool in the multiple ligament-injured knee sur-geon's tool box.

REVISION MULTIPLE LIGAMENT KNEE RECONSTRUCTION

Woodmass and colleagues[22] reported their outcomes after revisions of failed multiple ligament reconstruction surgery and showed that almost 50% of failures had an

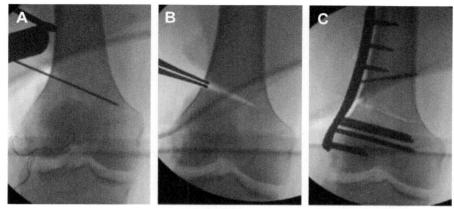

Fig. 2. Intraoperative fluoroscopy images of lateral opening wedge varus producing osteotomy. (*A*) Guide pin drilled through lateral distal femur. (*B*) Opening lateral wedge without compromising medial femoral cortex. (*C*) Bone grafting the open wedge and fixation.

unaddressed concomitant pathology. Osteotomy was required in 4 patients (17.4%) to treat coronal malalignment (defined as >5°), and realignment osteotomy was performed in a staged fashion. Overall, good clinical results and moderate functional results were observed at a mean follow-up 7.5 years. Based on their results, they proposed a treatment algorithm for the management of the failed multiple ligament reconstruction patient. The algorithm recommends a staged realignment procedure if coronal malalignment greater than 5° is present.

COMBINED PROCEDURES

In combined realignment and ligament reconstruction procedures, the ligament reconstruction can be performed at the same time as the osteotomy, or deferred. In

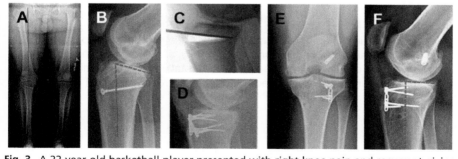

Fig. 3. A 22-year-old basketball player presented with right knee pain and recurrent giving way episodes. Surgical history consisted of 3 failed ACL reconstructions, and physical examination demonstrated high-grade Lachman and pivot shift. (*A*) AP radiograph showing normal coronal alignment. (*B*) Lateral radiograph showing increased posterior tibial slope of 25°. Additional computed tomography (CT) and MRI findings were large bony tunnels defects, medial meniscus deficiency, and lateral meniscus radial tear. A t2-stage revision was decided. The first stage included anterior proximal tibial closing wedge osteotomy, tunnel bone grafting, and lateral meniscus repair, and the second stage included ACL revision and medial meniscus transplantation. (*C*) Intraoperative fluoroscopy showing opening of anterior wedge. (*D*) Lateral radiograph after the first stage. (*E*) AP radiograph after the second stage. (*F*) Lateral radiograph after the second stage showing corrected posterior tibial slope of 7°.

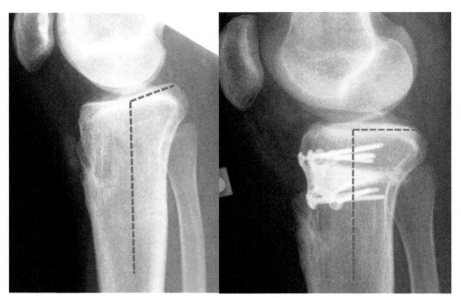

Fig. 4. Anterior opening-wedge high tibial osteotomy to increase posterior slope. On the left, preoperative lateral radiograph with negative posterior tibial slope. On the right, postoperative lateral radiograph with posterior tibial slope of 0°.

some cases ligament reconstruction is not necessary after the osteotomy, as sufficient stability, functionality, and pain reduction are achieved with the realignment procedures only.[23]

SUMMARY

Limb realignment in the coronal and sagittal planes must be carefully evaluated and treated in the setting of complex knee instability. Isolated soft tissue procedures are prone to failure if significant malalignment, deformity, and thrust are ignored. In select cases, osteotomy can lead to restored mechanical stability, optimal joint load distribution, improved survival of simultaneous soft tissue procedures, and better patient outcomes.

REFERENCES

1. Veltri DM, Warren RF. Operative treatment of posterolateral instability of the knee. Clin Sports Med 1994;13(3):615–27.

2. Noyes FR, Simon R. The role of high tibial osteotomy in the anterior cruciate ligament-deficient knee with varus alignment. In: DeLee JC, Drez D, editors. Orthopaedic sports medicine. Principles and practice. Philadelphia: WB Saunders; 1994. p. 1401–43.

3. Chang A, Hayes K, Dunlop D, et al. Thrust during ambulation and the progression of knee osteoarthritis. Arthritis Rheum 2004;50(12):3897–903.

4. Southam BR, Colosimo AJ, Grawe B. Underappreciated factors to consider in revision anterior cruciate ligament reconstruction: a current concepts review. Orthop J Sports Med 2018;6(1). 2325967117751689.

5. Won HH, Chang CB, Je MS, et al. Coronal limb alignment and indications for high tibial osteotomy in patients undergoing revision ACL reconstruction. Clin Orthop Relat Res 2013;471(11):3504–11.

6. Cantin O, Magnussen RA, Corbi F, et al. The role of high tibial osteotomy in the treatment of knee laxity: a comprehensive review. Knee Surg Sports Traumatol Arthrosc 2015;23(10):3026–37.

7. Noyes FR, Barber-Westin SD, Hewett TE. High tibial osteotomy and ligament reconstruction for varus angulated anterior cruciate ligament-deficient knees. Am J Sports Med 2000;28(3):282–96.

8. Giffin JR, Shannon FJ. The role of the high tibial osteotomy in the unstable knee. Sports Med Arthrosc Rev 2007;15(1):23–31.

9. Noyes FR, Barber-Westin SD, Albright JC. An analysis of the causes of failure in 57 consecutive posterolateral operative procedures. Am J Sports Med 2006; 34(9):1419–30.

10. Tischer T, Paul J, Pape D, et al. The impact of osseous malalignment and realignment procedures in knee ligament surgery: a systematic review of the clinical evidence. Orthop J Sports Med 2017;5(3). 2325967117697287.

11. Phisitkul P, Wolf BR, Amendola A. Role of high tibial and distal femoral osteotomies in the treatment of lateral-posterolateral and medial instabilities of the knee. Sports Med Arthrosc Rev 2006;14(2):96–104.

12. Agneskirchner JD, Hurschler C, Wrann CD, et al. The effects of valgus medial opening wedge high tibial osteotomy on articular cartilage pressure of the knee: a biomechanical study. Arthroscopy 2007;23. https://doi.org/10.1016/j.arthro.2007.05.018.

13. Cameron JC, Saha S. Management of medial collateral ligament laxity. Orthop Clin North Am 1994;25(3):527–32.

14. Hetsroni I, Lyman S, Pearle AD, et al. The effect of lateral opening wedge distal femoral osteotomy on medial knee opening: clinical and biomechanical factors. Knee Surg Sports Traumatol Arthrosc 2014;22(7):1659–65.

15. Sherman SL, Thompson SF, Clohisy JCF. Distal femoral varus osteotomy for the management of valgus deformity of the knee. J Am Acad Orthop Surg 2018; 26(9):313–24.

16. Getgood A, LaPrade RF, Verdonk P, et al. International meniscus reconstruction experts forum (IMREF) 2015 consensus statement on the practice of meniscal allograft transplantation. Am J Sports Med 2017;45. https://doi.org/10.1177/0363546516660064.

17. Hsu AC, Tirico LEP, Lin AG, et al. Osteochondral allograft transplantation and opening wedge tibial osteotomy: clinical results of a combined single procedure. Cartilage 2017. https://doi.org/10.1177/1947603517710307.

18. Giffin JR, Stabile KJ, Zantop T, et al. Importance of tibial slope for stability of the posterior cruciate ligament deficient knee. Am J Sports Med 2007;35(9):1443–9.

19. Giffin JR, Vogrin TM, Zantop T, et al. Effects of increasing tibial slope on the biomechanics of the knee. Am J Sports Med 2004;32(2):376–82. https://doi.org/10.1177/0363546503258880.

20. Robin JG, Neyret P. High tibial osteotomy in knee laxities: concepts review and results. EFORT Open Rev 2016;1(1):3–11. Available at: http://www.ncbi.nlm.nih.gov/pmc/articles/PMC5367616/.

21. Wang JH, Bae JH, Lim HC, et al. Medial open wedge high tibial osteotomy. Am J Sports Med 2009;37(12):2411–8. Available at: http://journals.sagepub.com/doi/full/10.1177/0363546509341174.

22. Woodmass JM, O'Malley MP, Krych AJ, et al. Revision multiligament knee reconstruction: clinical outcomes and proposed treatment algorithm. Arthroscopy 2018;34(3):744.e3.

23. Arthur A, LaPrade RF, Agel J. Proximal tibial opening wedge osteotomy as the initial treatment for chronic posterolateral corner deficiency in the varus knee: a prospective clinical study. Am J Sports Med 2007;35(11):1844–50.

Printed and bound by CPI Group (UK) Ltd, Croydon, CR0 4YY

08/05/2025

01864691-0007